BODY & SOUL: NARRATIVES
Edited by Allison Crawford, Rex Kay, Allan Peterkin, Robin Roger, and Ronald Ruskin, with Aaron Orkin

'*Body & Soul* tosses a rescue rope across the growing chasm between science and humanism. These poignant and powerful pieces speak volumes about the healing properties of narrative medicine from the perspective of health care professions and patients as well as their families. This is medical humanities at its finest.'
Barbara Sibbald, *Humanities Editor,* Canadian Medical Association Journal, *and author of* The Book of Love: Guidance in Affairs of the Heart

'*Body & Soul* comes from a brilliant collective of health professionals and patients whose insights are intellectual, humane and literary. I have watched the editors work their magic for years and there is no more sensitive and stimulating group I know now working in Canadian literature.'
Antanas Selekas, *Director of Humber School for Writers, and author of* Underground

'*Body & Soul* makes the distinct contribution of offering multiple perspectives on illness and care. In these pages, we hear the voices of patients, their families and friends, and those who offer professional care. This collection will be of particular value to teachers of healing arts and reflective practice. No other volume I know covers such a broad spectrum of experiences, each richly articulated.'
Arthur W. Frank, *author of* At the Will of the Body, The Wandering Storyteller, The Renewal of Generosity, *and* Letting Stories Breathe

Illness affects us all; we are called on to support and care for loved ones who face health challenges, and in turn, we encounter our own physical and emotional frailties when our health declines. *Body & Soul* features inspiring and award-winning fiction, essays, memoirs, poetry, photography, and visual art on the universal themes of wellness, treatment, and healing.

Told from the points of view of patients, practitioners, caregivers, families, and friends, *Body & Soul* provides a powerful literary perspective on how we are challenged, bewildered, changed, and uplifted by our encounters with change, illness, and disease. Readers will appreciate the richness, depth, and diversity of these healing stories and will become motivated to generate and share their own transformative narratives.

Together with the online discussion guide (providing questions relating to selected pieces in the anthology), *Body & Soul* is an ideal text for courses and support groups as well as individual reflection. Students and practitioners from all clinical disciplines and scholars in the humanities and social sciences will find this text invaluable.

A link to the online discussion guide is available at utppublishing.com/Body-and-Soul-Narratives-of-Healing-from-Ars-Medica.html.

ALLISON CRAWFORD, MD, REX KAY, MD, ALLAN PETERKIN, MD, ROBIN ROGER, MA, and RONALD RUSKIN, MD, founded *Ars Medica: A Journal of Medicine, the Arts, and Humanities* in 2006. AARON ORKIN, MD, joined the editorial team for this book in 2010.

Body & Soul

Narratives of Healing from Ars Medica

Edited by Allison Crawford, Rex Kay, Allan Peterkin, Robin Roger, and Ronald Ruskin, with Aaron Orkin

UNIVERSITY OF TORONTO PRESS

Toronto Buffalo London

© University of Toronto Press 2012
Toronto Buffalo London
www.utppublishing.com
Printed in the U.S.A.

Reprinted 2014

ISBN 978-1-4426-1290-7 (paper)

∞

Printed on acid-free paper

Library and Archives Canada Cataloguing in Publication

Body & Soul : narratives of healing from Ars Medica / edited by Allison Crawford ... [et al.].

Includes bibliographical references.
ISBN 978-1-4426-1290-7

1. Canadian literature (English) – 21st century. 2. Medicine – Literary collections. I. Crawford, Allison II. Title: Body and soul. III. Title: Ars medica.

PS8237.M43B63 2011   C810.8'03561   C2011-906635-1

University of Toronto Press acknowledges the financial assistance to its publishing program of the Canada Council for the Arts and the Ontario Arts Council.

Canada Council for the Arts **Conseil des Arts du Canada**   **ONTARIO ARTS COUNCIL CONSEIL DES ARTS DE L'ONTARIO**

University of Toronto Press acknowledges the financial support of the Government of Canada through the Canada Book Fund for its publishing activities.

Contents

User's Guide   ix

General Introduction   3

Part 1: Patients

Introduction to Part 1   7

1 As One Might Expect   9
     William Bradley
2 Hands: A Suite of Stories   11
     Linda E. Clarke
3 Prenatal Exam   18
     Sarah Cross
4 Sunday Nights at the Shangri-La   20
     Cindy Dale
5 A Picture Made of Sound   30
     Anne Elliott
6 Centre of Dread   34
     Faye George
7 At Thirteen, Asthmatic / Medicine Pudding / First Day Home from the Hospital   38
     John Grey
8 Daughter Cells   41
     Jessica Handler
9 BSE   49
     Alison Hauch
10 Things Taken   55
     Isabel Hoskins
11 Pain Scale   61
     Paul Hostovsky
12 Seeing the Heart   63
     Catherine Jagoe

13 Matter and Energy   65
   Lorie Kolak
14 My Little Heart Attack   74
   Tom Lombardo
15 The Eighth Day   75
   Michael Constantine McConnell
16 Life Study   82
   Helen McLean
17 Second Sight   91
   Helen McLean
18 Lethargy, Resulting from the Sudden Extinction of Light / Swallows   98
   Mary O'Donoghue
19 On the Loss and Reconstruction of a Self   101
   Menorah Lafayette-Lebovics Rotenberg
20 The Cure of Metaphor   108
   Kenneth Sherman
21 Kasabach-Merrit Syndrome   110
   Heather Spears
22 Inadequacy of Impotence   113
   George J. Stevenson
23 Diabetes: My Body Says "Fall"   114
   Heather L. Stuckey
24 Care for the Patient   116
   Yvonne Trainer
25 I, Michael   118
   Christopher Willard

Part 2: Family and Friends

Introduction to Part 2   125

26 Drawing Insulin   127
   Anonymous

27 Days and Nights in NICU   130
     Christine Benvenuto
28 Eden and I Are Playing Go Fish   136
     Susie Berg
29 Palliation   137
     Pat Cason
30 All Out of Funny in Crystal Lake, California   143
     Stephan Clark
31 911   149
     Diane Foley
32 Stoma   154
     Kathie Giorgio
33 Unpacking My Daughter's Library   161
     Joan Givner
34 My Father's Polio   168
     Patricia F. Goldblatt
35 Lie Down   176
     Katherine Govier
36 Friendship Bracelets   182
     Jon Hunter
37 Hope from a Distance   185
     Nigel Leaney
38 Something Happened   192
     Jane Martin
39 The Right Thing to Say   196
     Kathy Page
40 Second Round   204
     Nancy Richler
41 On Different Hospital Floors   211
     Nicholas Samaras
42 The Alzheimer's Man   213
     Alan Steinberg
43 The Second Parlour   215
     Anne Marie Todkill
44 The Wong-Baker Scale   220
     Gina P. Vozenilek

45 Denial   226
   Gina Wilch and Ruby Roy

Part 3: Practitioners

Introduction to Part 3   231

46 Accident Room   233
   Jay Baruch
47 Tale of a T-Shirt   244
   Susan Croft
48 The Texture of a Word   251
   Ian G. Dorward
49 Table of Unidentified Contents   254
   Doug Guildford
50 Figuring the Ground   257
   Pam Hall
51 Refugees in Southeast Asia   259
   J. David Holbrook
52 Mid-winter Night / Summer Party   267
   Jill Leahman
53 On Pathography   269
   Robert Maunder
54 Elysium   276
   Pamela Stewart
55 First Day on the Wards   284
   Eileen Valinoti
56 On Call   290
   Paul Whang
57 Making Images   302
   Arthur Robinson Williams

User's Guide

This section provides a guide to readers looking for specific content within this volume. It is intended to help identify collections of pieces that address similar themes, events, conditions or experiences. Under each theme, corresponding pieces are identified by the author's surname and page number. This is by no means an exhaustive or comprehensive guide; the selections below have been categorized by the editors to guide and inspire readers and to make it easier for readers to find the pieces they might be looking for. This is merely a schematic, one of the many ways of reading and approaching these texts, but it is not the only way. We have categorized according to our own readings and impressions; the idiosyncrasies of this guide may serve as an avenue for exploration and discussion. There is no right way to read this literature; there is perhaps no wrong way to read it either.

Children & Parenting

Patients
Grey, 38
Hoskins, 55
O'Donoghue, 98

Family & Friends
Anonymous, 127
Berg, 136
Clark, 143
Foley, 149
Givner, 161
Goldblatt, 168
Vozenilek, 220
Wilch and Roy, 226

Practitioners
Croft, 244

Chronic Illness & Aging

Patients
Hauch, 49
Kolak, 65
McConnell, 75
McLean, 82, 91
Rotenberg, 101
Stuckey, 114
Willard, 118

Family & Friends
Anonymous, 127
Goldblatt, 168
Samaras, 211
Steinberg, 213

Death & Dying

Patients
Bradley, 9
Handler, 41
Willard, 118

Family & Friends
Cason, 137
Givner, 161
Govier, 176
Hunter, 182
Martin, 192
Samaras, 211
Todkill, 215

Practitioners
Dorward, 251
Stewart, 276

Mental Health

Patients
Dale, 20
O'Donoghue, 98
Rotenberg, 101
Trainer, 116

Family & Friends
Foley, 149
Leaney, 185

Practitioners
Stewart, 276
Williams, 302

Pregnancy & Childbirth

Patients
Cross, 18
Spears, 110

Family & Friends
Benvenuto, 130
Page, 196
Samaras, 211

Professionals, Professionalism & Caring Practices

Patients
Clarke, 11
Elliott, 30

Family & Friends
Benvenuto, 130
Vozenilek, 220

Practitioners
Baruch, 233
Holbrook, 259
Maunder, 269
Valinoti, 284
Whang, 290

Symptoms & Procedures

Patients
Elliott, 30
George, 34
Grey, 38
Handler, 41
Hostovsky, 61
Jagoe, 63
Lombardo, 74
McConnell, 75
McLean, 82, 91
Rotenberg, 101
Sherman, 108
Stevenson, 113

Family & Friends
Giorgio, 154
Goldblatt, 168
Richler, 204
Steinberg, 213
Vozenilek, 220

Practitioners
Dorward, 251
Hall, 257
Leahman, 267

BODY & SOUL

General Introduction

In 2006, *Ars Medica: A Journal of Medicine, the Arts and Humanities*, was created in order to broaden and deepen the healthcare debate here in Canada and worldwide. The goal was to move from the usual clinical and pragmatic descriptions of healthcare encounters to the richly humane, by adding a narrative dimension to portrayals of the universal experience of illness, treatment and healing. The founding editors believed that a core, curative aspect of recovery is the relationship between the patient and the practitioner, and that this relationship is best understood when all parties in the process tell stories from their own perspectives. *Ars Medica* has become an important literary venue for the telling and honouring of those tales.

As you will see in this anthology, the richness of the contributions confirms our original conviction and strengthens it. What follows is a selection of some of our favourite pieces, but by no means all of them. After half a decade, we have an embarrassment of riches.

A question we continue to ask ourselves at *Ars Medica* is: What can patients and health practitioners do to address the growing divide between science and humanism? Storytelling is actually a great place to start. A shared assumption among the editors of *Ars Medica* is that good (i.e., curious, critical) readers make good healers and that medical tales aren't only told on the page, but also in our offices. Attentive reading of illness narratives and attentive listening to accounts of illness in our clinics are variations of the same skill. T.S. Eliot once said that we read many books because we cannot know enough people. This is as true for patients as it is for health practitioners whatever the discipline. It is helpful for both parties to gain exposure to each other's stories, so that clinicians are mindful of what it means to be a patient and patients are mindful of the challenges faced by the people trying to heal them. The partnership is strengthened from both directions.

That is why we have selected pieces told from the perspectives of everybody involved in our health community: practitioners, students, patients, their family and friends and professional artists and medicine watchers, all of whom bear witness to an encounter with healthcare. Our strategy is to help develop narrative competence, the ability to receive, comprehend, interpret and co-construct stories, for all parties involved, in the pursuit of health and wellness. For those of us who are clinicians, the advantage of discovering literary pieces together is that we can identify and discuss human predicaments as a sort of proxy for clinical situations without the pressure to rush off to fix things instead of reflecting on them. Practitioners are allowed to be moved and to appreciate the text, thus engaging both sides of our brain. We can judge, dislike, dismiss or be intrigued, attracted or confused by certain characters because literature like nothing else allows each of us to imagine and try to understand the Other. All readers of fine literature, whether medical professionals or laypeople, can experience the beauty and ambiguity of language, stretch their world view and become more complete, engaged citizens in a complex, storied world. Not only does this enrich life, it makes for a more effective and communicative engagement between practitioner and patient when the encounter eventually does take place.

A growing body of research has demonstrated that exposure not only to literature but to the fine arts, history, philosophy and anthropology broadens our cultural competence and encourages a linking of both cognitive and affective approaches to the task of caring for others. Poets, musicians and artists have been contemplating suffering since time immemorial and still have much to teach us. They give clinicians permission to rediscover the art in what they do every day and to fully imagine what makes that work beautiful and fundamentally human.

True healers have always used images and texts to help patients find the way. And patients have always sought to heal themselves through creative expression as well as through clinical encounters. And when health is restored, the experience of illness is metabolized through integrating a story about the event into one's life history and sense of self. Symptom, onset, treatment, recovery and loss each have their own story, giving rise to an infinite supply of meaningful narratives that speak to all of us as fully embodied creatures.

When we embarked on the creation of *Ars Medica* the many great literary works about medicine, health, the body and its vicissitudes convinced us that there were more stories to be told in our own communities, if a venue could be created for them. We have been deeply gratified, not only to bring these to light in the pages of *Ars Medica*, but also to interact with our contributors as editors during the acceptance and revision process. We have learned first-hand that in addition to reading narratives, assisting in the process of honing and perfecting them is a powerful and inspiring experience for editors and aids our understanding of what the journal should be. This act of co-construction has been genuinely healing. We hope that *Body & Soul*, as well as the journal itself, will become a part of your healing and reflective practice, whether you are a care provider, recipient or both.

Allan Peterkin, MD
Robin Roger, MA

Part 1: Patients

Introduction

Sooner or later, in the cycle of life from childhood to old age, we become patients. Existentially there appears to be no escape from this fate—it is an inevitable part of our most personal human drama that one day we experience suffering in our bodies and minds, as well as the suffering of friends and loved ones. Indeed, the word patient derives from the Latin verb patior (to suffer), offering us a double meaning, to suffer and experience pain, and patience, the bearing of suffering with calmness, self-control and tolerance.

Why write about suffering—what possible benefit is it to know or feel another's pain? Who is patient enough to read such stories?

The answer seems straightforward—the writing and telling of patients' stories shares and ennobles their struggles, de-mystifies the isolated unrecorded moment, expands the awareness and empathic response of others, and provides a vital dynamic link that unites the patient to the rest of the observing world. The stories, poems and art offer the patient an opportunity to rework and re-fashion their illness into a creative experience that itself offers a form of healing. To the curious (and anxious) reader, understanding the plight of others draws one more intimately to the other and to one's self.

These selected stories in the anthology seek to illuminate the patient's confrontation with illness in their personal narrative—for example, a gifted visual artist losing the vivid sense of colour undergoes eye surgery, a patient struggles with an unresponsive physician and post-surgical pain, a bereaved surviving sibling recounts the last seconds of a brother's life, a grieving sister puzzles over the flawed genes that claimed her two sisters, a young man chronicles his recovery from a paralyzing illness.

As readers we respond to the critical life dilemmas of these patients to become compassionately involved with the meaning and impact of illness. Compassion or passion, that is, being acted upon to produce emotion is yet another derivation from the Latin word for suffering.

This anthology welcomes the reader to be touched and explore each story.

Ronald Ruskin, MD

As One Might Expect

William Bradley

The nun came in the afternoon. At least, I think she was a nun. Although she didn't wear a habit, she had rosary beads, and a tiny plastic statue of the Blessed Virgin that she gave to me. She was a small, dark-skinned, soft-spoken woman with a thick accent, but I understood her question, pronounced softly that first day in her unidentifiable accent: "Would you like me to pray with you?" On the surface, it seemed like a silly question to ask a twenty-two-year-old guy in a hospital bed, with tubes sticking in his chest, a guy without energy, motivation, or hair. Groggy, confused, with a sense that things had once been better. Did I want to pray?

They say there are no atheists in foxholes or on crashing planes. I doubt there are too many in bone marrow transplant centres, either. And even if I were an atheist (and I wasn't—I was simply a Catholic with agnostic leanings), would I really want to take the chance and refuse such a pleasant woman who—maybe, probably—was a bride of Christ? What if Christ were watching, making sure people weren't rude to one of his brides? Ready to put a divine smackdown on anyone who was. Maybe that wasn't likely, but still, what reason was there not to pray?

My mother was sitting in the chair off to the side of the bed, looking up from her book, watching me from behind her bifocals. That was a reason to decline. My mother had never had much use for religion. My father insisted on going to midnight Mass, on saying grace, on rubbing water sent by relatives who had visited Lourdes on the lump that I'd found in my neck. My mother did not seem to care one way or another.

My mother was an English teacher, though, and I was training to become one. And although we had different interests and aesthetics, one thing that all lovers of literature have in common is an aversion to cliché. My mother liked originality, and I preferred ironic detachment. Really, what could be more clichéd than the cancer patient finding God? The smug Cathnostic begging to be saved, promising to be a better person if only this nightmare would end.

Ridiculous. Horrible. Daytime Emmy Award–winning shit, to be a stock character, as boring as an Amy Grant record being played at Kathy Lee Gifford's house. Could be a fate worse than death, I imagine.

Could be.

But probably not.

My mother didn't say anything, returning her focus to the novel in front of her, as I sat up from under the hospital bed's thin white sheets and let the nun—probably, she was a nun—take my hands. She closed her eyes; I closed mine as well. The words she spoke were low and in that heavy accent, but I made out the relevant parts. Prayers mostly tend to sound alike.

William Bradley's work has appeared or is forthcoming in the Missouri Review, Flashquake, *the* Snake Nation Review, *and the* Bellevue Literary Review. *In the fall he will begin teaching creative writing at Florida Atlantic University.*

Hands: A Suite of Stories

Linda E. Clarke

It is December and cold—bright but cold. Walking to the medical school I breathe deeply, relishing the quiver of excitement that traces down my spine: nervous tinged with fear. It is the end of my first term as artist-in-residence at the medical school, where I am a writer and a storyteller. This morning I am going to look at the bodies in the anatomy lab for the first time: totally normal to be excited, to be nervous. I'm wearing my grungy clothes—prepared as Fiona told me to be, for being bathed in the smells of chemicals and the bodies that are steeped in them.

Fiona, a second-year medical student, is a wonderful guide into this place. She is waiting for me and we make friendly chatter as we enter the building and ride the elevator to the anatomy lab, on the fourteenth floor. I am thankful that it is Christmas break—the building is quiet and there is little chance I will meet anyone I know and have to explain myself. This going to look at bodies feels secretive, an act that is kept in the shadows.

The elevator deposits us on the silent fourteenth floor. We exit and stand for just a moment by the display cases against the wall outside the entrance to the lab. The cases are benign, containing artifacts from anatomy endeavours of times gone by. Over Fiona's shoulder I can look into the lab, and I begin to make out rows of figures, white-draped and wrapped in plastic, some of them zipped into white bags that look, for a brief moment, like overstuffed garment bags. The shapes swim into clear focus and it dawns on me that they are bodies—rows of them, waiting for us. I swallow the nervousness before it carries me back onto the elevator and out into the winter sunshine. I don't dare breathe too deeply now.

We take off our winter coats and don white lab coats. Fiona shows me how to wash up and how to take care around these bodies, these men and women. She checks the tags on some of the bags—I have asked her to show me the body of a woman first. Finding one, Fiona carefully unzips the bag, exposing the woman's body wrapped in yellowed and damp gauze. She unwraps the cloth, leaving one layer covering the face, and I catch my breath. Tears prick at my eyes. I am alarmed and thrilled. This woman, such a solid, hulking presence, is exposed for us to see.

We spend some time looking at this woman, and inside her. The woman's chest wall has been cut away and one of her lungs has been excised. Her body cavity is wondrous, and once I stop thinking about the face I will not look at, I feel the trill of excitement calming down.

Her right hand rests at her side, as it would if she were asleep. It too is wrapped in gauze. Fiona tells me that, when the students first start looking at the bodies, they are warned that the hand is often the part of the body that upsets people—it is so highly personal. Fiona unwraps the hand as though it were made of glass and lays it down again. She steps back for me to see. This hand has been professionally dissected—the skin on the back of it has been peeled away from the wrist to the knuckles. Inside I can see the lacework of blood vessels and sinew and fine bones. The fingers, her fingers, are intact, and I notice that her nails are beautifully manicured and that there is a sprinkle of age spots dotting the flesh on the back of her fingers, or maybe they are freckles.

Four years earlier, in the dead of winter, I became very sick. It had been coming on for months, and the pain clamped down as the cold tightened its grip on the city. By day the light hurt my eyes and I could do little but wait for the dark of the night. Every evening, after I washed the dishes, I put on my heavy winter clothes. I layered on a sweater and my warmest thick coat, my wool socks and my big boots; then I pulled on a hat and stepped outside onto our back stoop. That was a season of heavy snow, and most evenings our backyard shone purple under the high winter moon. Time and time again, I walked out into the middle of that yard and turned to face the house. Then I bent to the task of making snowballs, building a pile of them, a pyramid beside me. Taking a deep breath, I threw them, one at a time, as hard as I could, against the brick wall of the house. I loved the thud as they hit the brick and the pattern of snow that would dot the wall as my pile dwindled. And how well I remember that with each throw I tried to throw away the pain that was becoming so much part of me; I wished myself into those snowballs and, with what energy I could find, tried to heave all that pain and suffering and worry and fear and powerlessness against the wall. When the snowballs were finished, I lay down in the snow and breathed up into the stars that shone crystal bright in the inky sky above me. I remember watching the cloud of my breath float into that sky and I remember longing to breathe myself and all that pain away.

And when I was cold, I went back into the warm house, where I took off my heavy winter coat and hat and wool socks. I walked into the living room where James was sitting on the couch, waiting for me. He opened his arms to me and I climbed into his embrace where he would rock me to sleep. Time and time again.

And I remember going to see a doctor whose promise I had trusted, the promise he made to accompany me through whatever was, as he said, "going on." I remember sitting across from him at the great sea of his desk and feeling choked as he told me that he thought I was "depressed." "Depressed?" after only one visit and the standard battery of tests. He spread his great hands in front of him—palms open.

"On this hand," he said to me, showing me his left palm, "I think you are depressed. On this other hand," the right, "if you take antidepressants, we can keep looking to see if there is anything else wrong with you."

And I remember travelling early one morning, cold and grey, to see an ophthalmologist who had reluctantly agreed to see me as a favour to someone else. James drove and I rode beside him in the passenger seat, closing my eyes against the pain and trying hard to find the balance between optimism and realism.

I sat in the big chair while that doctor examined my eyes: dim lights and great big machines. He was so close to me I could smell his minty breath and see the whiskers on his closely shaven chin. I remember he wore a denim shirt, and cartoon figures cavorted on his tie. When he was finished the exam, he pushed away on his wheeled stool to flip the light back on. Then he wheeled back to me, close again. He began to snap his fingers, first his right hand, then his left, one after the other, and to fly them around between the two of us—close to his face, close to my face.

Snap Snap Snap

"What are you doing?" I asked.

Snap Snap Snap

"Killing flying monkeys," came the answer. My heart turned to ice.

Snap Snap Snap

"Do you see any flying monkeys?" he continued.

I shook my head, "No."

Snap Snap Snap

"And I don't see anything wrong with you." he replied, the flying monkeys coming to rest in his lap. And with that I was dismissed.

And I remember the technician's hands in the CT lab as she motioned abruptly for me to lie down on the narrow bench and handed me the blue paper shower cap to keep my hair at bay. I remember her hands, cool and long fingered, putting the Velcro strap across my forehead to keep me still.

And I remember her hands when the scan was finished (almost an hour later) and she reached to help me sit up and rested her hand on my shoulder and asked me, with a kind voice, if I was feeling all right. And then helped me out of the room, her hand on the small of my back, warm now. And I remember knowing then that she had seen something in my brain, because her hands were so suddenly kind and patient. And I swallowed that thought with the air I breathed and walked back out to James in the waiting room.

And three days later I remember my own hand gripping the receiver of the phone in the kitchen, white knuckled, listening to the doctor, my doctor, tell me that "they didn't find nothing," a double negative that made me sit down carefully on the floor while he told me what they found and what it might mean.

"Thank God," I said, "I didn't waste anyone's time."

And I remember the hand of my neurosurgeon when he snapped the film, MRI film now, into the light box in his office and pointed out the round shape, nestled in the centre of my brain. "That will have to come out," he said, and I remember his finger was long and dark against the light.

And then there were the healing hands of our neighbour lady who is a little witchy and full of spells from a lifetime of laying on of hands. She came over to the house the night before the surgery, and her touch was like oil on troubled seas, healing and calming. I remember sitting on the straight-backed chair, feeling foolish, until her hands touched me ever so gently, and her voice, wrapped in the softness of an Irish accent, quieted me down. She promised to come with us the morning of the surgery, to lay her hands on me before the procedure.

And there were the hands of the resident—a business-only-stiff-upper-lip woman of sharp edges and cold fingers whose job it was to put the great metal frame onto my head, whose fingers fixed the tiny screws through my scalp and into my skull. The small crackling sound of those screws going into my skull will stay with me forever.

I lived in the ICU for three weeks after surgery. In the early morning hours, when the lights were still dimmed, there came a dark shadow of a nurse. In those hours, her soft voice of chocolate and warm sugar reached for me in the depth of my sleep and drew me back into the unit. In her big hands she carried a basin of warm water, and from my drowsiness I would watch as she opened a bottle of lavender oil and dripped it—one, two, three times—into the warm water. She sang under her breath and spoke to me only occasionally as she reached with her brown velvet hands and pulled me to lean into her so she could untie my gown and wash me. I could feel her heart thrumming with the soft hymns that she was singing, hum halleluiah gentle. And her hands reached into that warm water, dipped a white cloth and wiped me clean: my face and my hands and up my arms, gentle dipping, hum halleluiah gentle, and my back and my breasts and under my arms. And when she was finished she wrapped me in a clean gown and she laid me down onto my pillow and I would tumble back into sleep.

Every word of this is true: once, in the ICU, I had this dream. I am, it seems, hanging onto a white rope ladder. It is a totally dark place, but warm and safe, not a place of fear. Close to me I can hear others, whispers around me. I look down and see the ladder stretching away beneath me into the darkness, and I look up and see that it reaches far above me as far as the eye can see.

My hands grip the rung at eye level, they are aching, burning, and I see that they are white-knuckled. My feet are tired, bare on the rung below. I breathe there, exhausted.

And then I hear a voice, a voice that tells me I can let go of the ladder if I want to. That I won't be hurt and I won't fall away but I will end up in a different place. Or, the voice tells me, I can choose to keep climbing. It's my choice. I hang there and long to float off into the darkness. But I reach up to the rung above me and pull myself higher.

And there were times I woke up from the sleep that held me close those first weeks and found James sitting beside my great high bed, his head bent as he read a book, one hand holding mine, and the warmth of his hand would lead me back to peaceful sleep.

And I remember my surgeon coming, as he so often did, to check on me. He stood beside my bed and softly called my name while he woke me up by gently, ever so gently, stroking my arm.

So much power in one hand.

And from my perch in the ICU I saw countless hands and opportunities to lay on hands and lost opportunities and hands as tools and hands as weapons. Hands carrying trays of food and drinks of water and medicine, hands checking lines and making notes, and hands holding the hands of loved ones. Missed chances and chances taken.

Oaxaca is in the southwest corner of Mexico. It sits at the head of a valley that is graced with ancient sites of the people who lived there thousands of years before the arrival of the Europeans. It is a wondrous place. In that place there is a millennia-old tradition of healers who use herbs and ritual to care for people who are ill, *curanderos*. Nine months after my surgery I packed up my life in Toronto and moved to Oaxaca, where James had been working since May. It had been planned many months before I took ill and was a goal for me to accomplish through the struggle to get well, my light at the end of the tunnel. I remember packing up my winter gear to be left behind in my parents' basement, and thinking on it, it is as though I really believed that somehow I could pack away the self that had been so sick and in so much pain and leave that person behind, buried in the midst of all that winter gear. But, of course, that wasn't to be—I carried myself with me to Oaxaca.

A month after my arrival there I met Alejandro: Alma, the boss's wife, told me he was a *curandero* who was good at treating pain. I agreed to see him. One grey December afternoon she brought Alejandro to the gate of our small bungalow. She introduced us to one another, telling me that he spoke some English and telling him, in Spanish of course, that I spoke some Spanish. I liked him right away: he was a compact handsome man with a shy smile. Alma left, and it was just the two of us. I invited Alejandro into our small home and closed the door.

Alejandro motioned for me to sit down at the table and he stood behind me. He managed to make himself understood and he explained that he was going to touch my head. I sat quietly. Even then I fervently hoped for a magic touch that would take the weight of my pain away from me. He put both of his hands on top of my head, his finger gently tracing the outline of the hole in my skull.

He asked me what had happened. *"¿Que paso aqui?"*

"Una cosa en mi cerebro, something in my head," I shyly said. *"Tengo un operation."* Very poor Spanish, meaning to say "I had an operation."

I melted at the words I was saying. I wanted so much for this man to know what had happened to me, I wanted him to carry it away.

He rested his hands there for a few moments. Then he walked around and sat down facing me, very close.

"Eres una cunadera, you are a healer." He told me. "I feel it very strongly."

"What do you mean?" I asked. My heart was thundering.

"I get a strong feeling that you are a healer," he said, "It is what you are to people."

"But I have a lot of pain," I told him, "and I don't know what to do to make it go away."

"You will heal yourself by telling your story to other people," he answered. "There is healing in the telling. And in telling other people your story, you will help them heal as well."

And so, with the flow of time, I came to be in the anatomy lab at the medical school, surrounded, on that bright cold winter morning, by the quiet dead. And standing there, I knew that each of their stories was written onto their very bodies, right into their very bones. I stepped closer to the woman's body and examined her hand, picking it up gently and running my fingers, ever so gingerly, along the lines of it, the hills and valleys. It is in the hand, I remember thinking, that all that is human is captured.

The stories of the health care community are a passion for Linda E. Clarke, writer and storyteller. As an artist and an educator, her work in health care humanities has spanned more than 20 years. Linda has performed, broadcast, and published widely. One way or another, she is full of stories.

Prenatal Exam

Sarah Cross

One: fundal height
as measured from pubic symphysis–
slowly unhooking–
to the uterine summit.
Normally unassuming organ:
spends most of its time
in unrequited preparation,
now a visceral tank pushing
toward the lungs.
Thirty-eight weeks at the xyphoid
before she drops.

Two: head engaged
deep in the pelvis,
a compact water acrobat
she is hanging,
ballotable, obliging,
feel for her back.

Three: fooled by the cord blood
at first, which is fast,
but rushing, not beating.
What goes on submerged
within that cavern of muscle?
Listen through the
gel-covered landscape,
spelunker-like
unrefined divination skills
search the heart.

Four: with no map suddenly
the sound comes through
at 153, right of the umbilicus:
unearthed sound reverberating
in the narrow room—
tiny motor, its reassuring speed.

Sarah Cross won the 24th Annual William Carlos Williams Poetry Competition and received honourable mention in the 12th Annual New Physician's Creative Arts Contest. She is guest editing a collection of poems for the Journal of Medical Humanities.

Sunday Nights at the Shangri-La

Cindy Dale

8:57 p.m. I log on, enter the chat room, no one's here. Type in *Hey*—to the void. Sarah's always here first, and that scares me. This is the third Sunday in a row she hasn't shown. Here's a girl who joined in religiously for fourteen weeks straight and suddenly she's gone. If this were AA, you could be certain she'd fallen off the wagon. But it's not AA, and well, damn it, I'm worried.

The trouble is I have no way of contacting her. I don't even know her last name, or where she lives. Somewhere in Montana, near Missoula maybe? Which is not necessarily a good thing, statistically speaking at least. You think of Montana as "Big Sky" country. You think of snow-peaked mountains and crystal-clear rivers and streams studded with silvery trout. You think of a place where there are more cows, deer, and elk than there are people. But Montana is also the state with the second-highest suicide rate per 100,000 population, sandwiched neatly between Nevada at #1 and Alaska at #3. Now those two you can understand, but Montana? Isn't it supposed to be God's country?

Sarah's brother Matt was one of those statistics five months ago. He shot himself through the head with his father's pistol, choosing the most popular route to the other side. He was nineteen years old and had just completed his freshman year at the University of Montana. He didn't leave a note, but then only 40 per cent of people do. You've got to wonder why. Wouldn't you want to get that final "fuck you" in before exiting stage left? Maybe you're too worried about messing that up, too. After all, chances are you aren't Shakespeare, and it's easy to imagine the authorities scrutinizing your misplaced commas, your errors in proper tense. But by the time they find your note, you're most likely newly past tense anyway so what the hell difference does it matter?

Sarah's fifteen. She's the only one left now. Her parents don't let her out of their sight, having curtailed even cheerleading practice. They're constantly asking how she's feeling. Hell, they've even removed the Aspirin from the medicine cabinet, just in case. Can you blame her for feeling like she's slowly going nuts?

Of course I understand. All of us here understand. Maybe we're the only ones who really do. I mean, we've all got these phantom siblings who are still hanging around the dinner table, despite their untimely demises. We've all got parents who—either jointly in a state of suicide-induced solidarity, speak to you in the imperial "we" or separately, the suicide being the final straw in what was probably a lousy marriage to begin with—watch over you, trying to do what all the damn therapists tell them to do, trying desperately to make you feel loved, determined not to miss those telltale signs a second time.

9:02 p.m. Hey—How's things? The words appear in bright green on my screen. Nicki's here.

Hey Nick, I type back. *Surviving.*

Nicki's twelve and lives in Shaker Heights. Her brother Gregg hung himself down in the basement on December 23. He was home from this famous boarding school for the Christmas break. According to Nicki, he never wanted to go there in the first place. But their father—this hotshot ESQ who was up for judge—had gone there, and Gregg had no choice, especially if he wanted to get into Yale a couple of years down the road, which is something his soon-to-be-Your-Honour never questioned.

Nicki was the one who found Gregg, although she's sure that wasn't his intention. He was hanging way back in the laundry room. She's convinced the ultimate *Fuck You* was intended for their mother, who was some kind of modern day Lady Macbeth when it came to cleanliness. *Out, damned spot!* Nicki never went back to the laundry room, but she was looking for her favourite pair of jeans that day—clean or dirty—and there you have it. Surprise! Gregg dangling, his face a sickly grey, his toes a mere two inches from the ground. Two goddamn inches. Might as well have been a mile.

Nicki's got two younger sisters—six and eight—but they don't get it. They still think Gregg's just back at boarding school again, that he'll be home when the Easter Bunny comes. Never mind the urn that's sitting on the mantelpiece. The girls—Alison and Madeline—weren't allowed at the funeral, so what do they know? To them, the golden urn is just another tennis/wrestling/track trophy waiting for Gregg to come and reclaim it.

9:04. Hey guys. No sign of Sarah? Brent's here.

His sister did the typical vodka-and-pill thing while away at school. Much cleaner that way, to do it away from home. Sure, you get the phone call but as Brent points out they'd been expecting it for years. She'd been through three plus years of the anorexia thing and had Emily Dickinson poems framed on her bedroom wall.

Nope. Nada. Rien. Zip. I'm worried, I type back.

Me, too. Nicki chimes in. *It's not like her.*

9:06. Sorry I'm late. Joshua joins in. *I was getting one of my 'we care for you so much' speeches. Tomorrow's his birthday and shit's weird around here.*

Joshua's brother Michael also took the gun route. There's some question about whether it really was a hunting accident, but no one believes that story. A slip of the finger on opening day. Happens all the time up in the Upper Peninsula where they live. Yeah, sure. But it makes for a much better story down at St. Joe's where he'd been an altar boy, taken his first communion, and God knows what else. That's what his parents tell everyone and that's the story Joshua is supposed to tell, too. Never mind that everyone knows better. I mean, there was the email Joshua got from Michael later that day. He showed his parents, but they never showed the authorities. It made things pretty damn clear.

Jesus, Josh. That sucks. How old would he have been? I forget, Nicki types.

Sixteen. Shit. It's just so fucking weird. My mom's making a fucking cake if you can believe it. Angel food because as she says, 'He's now with the angels.' The woman has absolutely lost it—

The first year is the worst, Brent jumps in. *Brianna's birthday was last month, and man it was rough. She would have been twenty. Ma didn't get out of bed for two days. Bri got some birthday cards from a couple of friends who still didn't know and it put ma over the edge.*

I can't help think about my own birthday and how it's basically screwed for life. Some say my story takes the cake. After all, I'm talking about my twin brother here—my identical twin brother. Larry, who was older than me by something like three minutes, taller than me by a quarter inch, the one who for some odd reason never needed braces. He off-ed himself by jumping from the Golden Gate Bridge during rush hour on the eve of our high school graduation. I truly challenge anyone to top that.

The bridge is the most popular jumping point in the world, by the way, having logged well over a thousand final exits since it opened up in 1937. It's a mere four seconds to reach the water and the average body hits at seventy-five miles per hour. Four seconds—one one thousand, two one thousand, three one thousand, four one thousand. Doesn't seem like much, but it must seem like a lifetime to the jumper and I can't help but wonder if Larry had second thoughts, if he glanced over towards Dad's office building and offered up a final little wave. Or flipped him the finger.

Here are a few facts about suicide for you:

Every eighteen minutes someone does themselves in in this country, the land of the free. Suicides outnumber homicides by five to three. The ratio of male to female is four to one. There are an estimated twenty-five attempts for every completion. I love that word. *Completion*. I guess you can't quite call it a success, can you?

Larry certainly completed. His jump stalled traffic for a good four hours on a Friday afternoon of a long holiday weekend. They stopped covering bridge suicides in the papers and on the TV a couple of years back, figuring it glorified the act, I suppose, giving the jumper the attention he or she was silently screaming out for. Somehow, word got out, though, and everyone knew it was Larry Grayburn, Winston and Lorraine's son. *Was he a troubled kid? Where there problems at home? Girl problems? Drugs?* Inquiring minds wanted to know. I mean, this was a kid who had everything—the proverbial golden boy—and he jumps off the goddamn Golden Gate Bridge. They've already established a scholarship in his name at the high school, making out like he's some kind of hero who died of cancer or in some James Dean–like car accident.

Good thing the yearbooks had already been printed. It was too late to slap his picture up front with a big "In Memoriam" banner, like they did for Stacy Clark and Jennifer Woodmere the year before after they died in that car crash that left J. J. Bonita in Superman's condition. I was looking at our yearbook just the other day, and there we are right next to each other in the senior section: Lawrence Grayburn and Lester Grayburn. I mean, who in hell names their kid Lester? If anything, I should have been the one to jump, what with a name like that.

She's turned the house into a fucking shrine, Joshua types, interrupting my reverie. *Everywhere you turn, there's Michael looking back at you. Even in the damn bathroom. I can't take a piss without him watching—*

It's the opposite here, Nicki types. *The pictures are all gone, like he never existed. But there are still all the trophies. And the urn. I mean, Gregg is sitting there right in the middle of the living room—*

My problem is, we're both in almost every picture. You can't get rid of one without the other, I jump in.

Yeah, I hadn't thought about that, Nicki types.

It's just weird, Joshua writes. *It's like picking a scab off a wound. Just when you're getting on with things, or trying to, she has to go and make an angel food cake—and there's no one who gets it—*

After it happens, no one knows what to say to you. Your parents are usually too numb from whatever drugs the doctors have got them on. Hell, they probably tried to make you take them, too. Your neighbours drop off cookies and casseroles, mumbling their condolences, glad to leave as quickly as they can. And your friends? They slap you on the back and say "Man—" Pop a beer for you. Say, "If there's anything you need—" But after the funeral where they turn up in force, you notice a gradual tapering off. It's almost as if you might be contagious, like it might run in the family or something. Could be their parents exerting pressure. "Be nice to poor Les, but hey—don't spend too much time with him, okay? Wouldn't you rather hang with Todd or Jack or David? I mean, they're nice boys—" Your parents will inevitably shuffle you off to some kind of shrink who will lean forward and say, "Tell me how you're feeling. Are you angry? It's okay to be angry—"

The truth is there's no one you can really talk about it with. I mean, I could have talked to Larry—but he's not here. You certainly can't talk to your parents, even if they're not anesthetized with drugs or scotch or whatever gets them through the night. Forget third parties—priests, guidance counsellors, shrinks you've only just met yesterday. And friends? Like I said, they weird out on you and do some sort of Houdini, maybe surfacing months later, acting as if nothing ever happened, which is even worse.

There are plenty of people around ready to take the blame, like your parents, or, hell, even you. It's never the dead kid's fault. Never mind that he is the one who pulled the trigger / took the pills / kicked back the stool / took the leap. It's never his fault. As a result, we've all got these siblings vying for retroactive sainthood.

I was going nuts. Then I found this place. Or, more accurately, this place found me. Word spreads about a suicide like Larry's. You start getting emails from people you don't even know, like Nicki. She's the cousin of a friend of a friend. She told me about the board. We call the place Sunday Nights at the Shangri-La because Sunday's the day of the week more youth suicides occur than any other and because this is the only place you can escape the stigma of being the surviving sibling. In fact, from our little club only Larry didn't do himself in on a Sunday. You've got to understand this is a very exclusive club. If your mom or your dad offed themselves, it doesn't count. Siblings who died of disease or accident or even drug overdose don't count either. You've got to be someone whose brother or sister pulled a Kevorkian way before his or her time. Now if Kurt Cobain had had a brother or a sister, we'd roll out the red carpet.

There's a mass tomorrow morning, and she's insisting I go, Joshua types. *I don't want to. Is that terrible? I just want to go to wrestling practice like usual and forget the whole damn thing—*

I know what you mean, Nicki types. *I'm dreading Matt's birthday. I really don't know. How it'll be. It's the Fourth of July. Fireworks and everything.*

Independence Day, I type. *What a joke. Guess he showed you all his independence, huh?*

You know, I wasn't really surprised, Nicki types. *I mean, I was but I wasn't. I've never said that before. He was so angry—angry at my dad, angry at the world—*

I was, I type. *Surprised, I mean. We'd been together that morning. At the graduation ceremony. He was talking about getting a keg for the party later. He was talking about Lydia, and how he couldn't believe she was going to LA to school, but how it didn't really matter—there were bound to be other girls at Cornell, he said. Not that it's Lydia's fault. It's not, but I didn't have a fucking clue. Not a fucking clue*—

Not me, Brent types. *I just wondered what took her so long. Jesus, I can't believe I said that. You know, she was so messed up for so long. But what bugs me is I don't know how she got that way. Was it one thing? Or just the culmination of lots of things? What happened to set her down that path*—

Yeah, I know what you mean, Nicki types. *You can't help but wonder if there was anything you could have done or said that would have made a difference.*

Yeah, I type. *I hear you*. I can't help thinking what would have happened if I'd gone with Larry that afternoon instead of with my friend Dylan. But who could have known? We were all headed the same place—Jackson's house—and we'd agreed to meet there at six. Who could have known that at 5:33 my identical twin brother would have parked his car in the middle of traffic—my mother's BMW, for Chrissake sake—and jumped off the goddamn bridge?

The experts will tell you the average youth suicide makes up his or her mind to commit the act within an hour of the actual attempt. Like Einstein once said, something about opportunity meeting the prepared mind. Still, I find it hard to believe Larry just suddenly decided to jump on his way home for whatever fucking reason. Because Lydia was going to UCLA? Because he'd been salutatorian and not valedictorian? I don't think so. Then I think, how could I have missed it? The signs. He'd given me this game ball that Steve Young had signed two days before. Told me to keep it, that he didn't need it anymore. I figured it was because he was going east to school and I was staying local, bound for Berkeley. But you know, that's one of the key signs. Giving away prized possessions. How the hell did I miss it? And what do I do with that football now?

Here are a few more facts about suicide for you. At some point in time, 53 per cent of high school students consider suicide. 53 fucking per cent. At any given point in time—I mean like right *now*—7 per cent of kids are thinking about it. Most teen suicides occur in the afternoon or early evening right in the kid's home, with the parents present. And like I said, Sundays—God's day, the day of rest—top the list.

Sunday nights tend to suck anyway, but hanging here helps. None of us have ever met. I have no idea if Nicki is pretty or if Josh has zits or whether Sarah has tits. It's irrelevant. We're all part of a club we never wanted to join. SOS. We're the true survivors of suicide, the ones who get left behind.

I've been coming to the club six months now. We don't email during the week. We don't have each other's phone numbers. But none of us would miss Sundays for anything, which is why Sarah being AWOL has got us all spooked.

You start with simple explanations. Maybe her grades were slipping and her parents cut off the Internet. Or maybe they went on some extended Caribbean vacation and Sarah just forgot to mention it when she was last here four weeks ago. Then your thoughts get darker. Maybe there was a car accident. Maybe she got diagnosed with some unpronounceable disease. Maybe—

Hey—Sarah's name appears on the screen.

Sarah??????????? We all type in simultaneously.

Yeah, it's me, Sarah types.

Where the hell you been girl? Nicki types.

God, we were worried, Joshua adds.

Yeah, we thought—you know, that something was seriously wrong. Or that you did something stupid, Brent adds.

I did, Sarah types.

What do you mean? I type.

I slit my wrists, Sarah types, adding a little smiley face with a frown.

Jesus Sarah! Why? Nicki asks.

I don't know. They were getting on me. My parents, I mean. They wouldn't let me go anywhere. And the kids at school . . . I don't know. It was like I was a leper or something—

But slitting your wrists? Come on girl, you can do better than that! You know only 15 per cent of those attempts work, Brent types.

Brent! It's Nicki again.

Hey, don't worry. Brent's right. I didn't really want to complete, to use the lingo. That's obvious. Even to me.

So why? I don't get it, Joshua types.

I don't know. It's weird, Sarah writes.

Yeah, go on, Josh says.

It was every cliché in the book. It was a Sunday night—the first night I didn't make it here. My parents were upstairs watching some movie of the week. I was down in the basement, working on my homework on the computer when, I don't know, the senselessness of it all came over me. I had to pee, and I went into the bathroom. I opened the medicine cabinet, and there was a package of razor blades behind this jar of hand lotion that they apparently missed when they suicide proofed the house—

So why weren't you logging on? Were you going to come that night? Here I mean,—I type.

Yeah, I was. After I finished my homework. It was doing a report on Montana. I was trying to find out what our state flower is—

And what is your state flower? Brent types. *Inquiring minds want to know <g>.*

The Bitterroot. Sarah types. *Nice name, huh?*

What's it look like? I type.

It's actually rather pretty—Kind of a purpley-pink. Grows close to the ground. Very hearty. A perennial.

Unlike our siblings. Brent types. *Sorry, it's all just so . . . . .*

Or maybe just like our siblings, Josh adds. *Forever with us, forever a piece of who we are, just because they're gone—*

So Sarah, what's it like? Those final moments? I type, hitting the send button before I can think about what I'm asking.

It's like they say in all the articles. You change your mind. You really do,— she writes.

Go on,—I type, suddenly wanting this insider's view of those final minutes. The damn experts I don't know about, but Sarah I trust.

You just change your mind. You want to live. You'd give anything to rewind, to go back and not do the stupid thing you've just done—I looked at the blood, and Jesus it was a lot of blood, and I thought 'I should get something to stop the bleeding.' The word tourniquet went through my mind, and I remember thinking, How do you spell that? Like it matters. Then I thought, 'I should call my mom or dad. I should scream. I started to get up, to go get someone, but I was dizzy, and the last thing I remember is going down, and seeing these flowers in my head—Bitterroot, I guess, blooming thick in a field, just like the poppies in The Wizard of Oz when Dorothy falls asleep—And I can't help but think about Larry. Larry parking the BMW *on the bridge and getting out. Standing at the edge, looking down. Maybe thinking about it right then, maybe not. Standing on the ledge, then leaping—One one thousand—feeling the liberation of free-fall, almost feeling like he can fly—two one thousand—that shadow of a doubt creeping in—three one thousand—then panic, thinking, What the fuck have I done? Why didn't anyone—Mom/Dad/Lydia/you—pick up on the fucking signals I was sending out? That final* SOS*—four one thousand, that millimetre before impact, cursing himself for this idiot act he has done, cursing all of us for the pedestal we put him on, so out of reach from the rest of the human race, cursing Sir Fucking Isaac Newton for discovering gravity in the first place—*

Cindy Dale's stories have appeared in literary journals, websites, and anthologies including Orchid, South Carolina Review, Zoetrope: All-Story Extra, *and* Potomac Review. *She lives on a barrier beach with her husband and two children.*

A Picture Made of Sound

Anne Elliott

TWO THINGS I fear becoming: (1) a hypochondriac, (2) a narcissist.

THE TECHNICIAN hands me a gown and looks down at my questionnaire clipboard. "You're young," she says. "Why you here?"

I'm a hypochondriac. "Family history," I say.

"More than one family member?"

"Yes."

She nods gravely. I look at the wall.

OH, I FORGOT, one more thing I fear becoming: (3) my mother.

I see her in a photograph, three years diagnosed, four years from dead. She, in a black formal gown with glass beads hanging lopsided across her front, earnest eyes peering up at her violin. The photos in sequence, a film strip. A long drag of the bow, a goofy grin. You can see the cacophony in the photo, the scratchy waves exiting the swirly soundholes, the almost-there pitch of the violin beginner. "My father never let me learn violin," she used to say. "He said the sound would drive him crazy."

"You're fifty years old," said her therapist. "He lives 500 miles away. He can't hear you from here."

I wasn't so sure. That noise had a way of hanging on the breeze.

"CAN I HAVE THAT?" I ask the X-ray technician. I collect pharmaceutical pens, use them to write in my notebook. "I'll trade you my Nexium for that Tamoxifen."

She shrugs, hands me the pen, wraps the lead apron around my middle. No, not pregnant, not even close. I wonder if all aprons are lead in some way, along with their strings, heavy and poisonous, sucking women and their offspring down to the bottom of the pool. The apron feels cool and good, though, this time, like a heavy heirloom quilt pinning me into bed.

"Hold still." I know the drill. Hold my breath, squish each side like blemished double-D cider apples, horizontal, then vertical, then angular, then a magnification of the area they seem to be watching.

A MONTH AFTER she died, I went to St. John the Divine, where a violinist played in the columbarium. I didn't want to interrupt, so I sat just outside the entrance, closed my eyes, and listened to his pure notes reverberate in the hollow marble room. Chaotic with its own past, notes remembered from the phrase just before, occasional dissonance, but mostly complementary harmonics, like the echo in a canyon or cistern.

The violinist stopped. I heard a man ask him why he played in the columbarium. Wasn't it obvious? "This is my best audience," said the musician, then bowed a long, high, naked open fifth, ending the conversation.

THE DOC ASKS if I can stay for ultrasound. Sure, I know the drill. I never see her, this doctor. She hides in a room full of slides and films and computer screens, like the Wizard of Oz. I re-gown and move to another room, where a new technician notices my notebook. "You're a writer?"

"Yeah, well, it's more of a hobby." My own scratchy sounds, practising, trying for something pure.

"Hobby, yeah, right." She can see right through my thick hide of self-effacement, straight to the part that takes itself too seriously. "My son is a writer." On the wall, a clear image of an unborn baby's face, a new soul, a picture made with sound. "I wanted my son to really do something with his writing, you know?" She squirts warm gel on my bare chest, begins the long process of looking for lesions. "He was so good in school, he got an award even from the *Daily News*."

"Wow." The light is dim. Her screen glows, echoing blue on the acoustic tile ceiling.

"But he had to get an MBA. I told him, OK, so if you are in business, at least try publishing, you know, surround yourself with what you love."

"That makes sense," I say.

"You write for a living?"

"No. I work in an office." Hardly surrounded with the stuff I love. "But if I didn't, I wouldn't be here."

"Insurance. True." I look up at her little screen, a black-and-white image of my own fat and blood.

"Anyway, who listens to their mother, right?" Then she blushes. She has seen my chart, knows mother is a weird word. A pause, as she types into her keyboard. "So, is your mother all right?"

"Nah, she's gone."

"I'm sorry."

I decide to keep it clinical. "Well, she was diagnosed in the eighties. A lot has changed." I think of my new pen: "Tamoxifen—that wasn't around yet."

"Yes, and the screening tools," she lightens up. "Wow. I got into this field just as it was exploding, about ten years ago. I got to see some of the miracles happen." She glides the sensor over my skin, shooting sound into my body. "You know, it was a woman engineer who figured out how to use harmonics. It's chaotic, you know, the way the sound echoes back. Used to be you'd get only a fuzzy picture. But she figured out how to analyze the chaos, so now we can even tell what kind of tissue we're looking at." Her eyes bright, echoing the harmonics on the screen, she loves her work, is surrounded by what she loves. "Like here," she clicks a pointer at a dark mass, "now we can tell this is just a cyst. No cutting."

"No unnecessary radiation."

"Exactly. And check this out: a woman invented this too. See, the machine gives off hot air. So they put this sleeve here for the gel, so the machine just warms it up. A man wouldn't've come up with that. It's too practical."

Mom used to say things like that. Irritating, sometimes, but not always. Some kind of warm gel is welling up in my solar plexus. I swallow it back down.

"The things we women go through," says the technician, as she starts in on the other side.

I think of Dad, stroking Mom's bald head, sometimes for more than an hour, to lull her to sleep. Going through something too.

The technician stops. "Check this out: see this thing moving here?"

I see it. I feel it. It's the edge of my nervous heart.

"Pericardium," she says.

"Oh." I knew it had a better name.

THE UNIVERSITY where Mom worked has an engineering scholarship in her name, for minorities and women, under-represented in the field. This year it went to a gal who plays violin in her spare time. I wonder what miracles she will witness. Or engineer.

I think of her, this stranger, her future facilitated by my mother's lack thereof, as I put my clothes back on and walk into the midtown evening. Against the hard city harmonics, honks and sirens, the hypochondriac pipes up: another year clear! The narcissist is almost disappointed: an illness could be my ticket out of the office and into my ready notebook. Think of the material!

And Mom, she's quiet, for the moment. I think she's busy. It's just another day. Maybe she's practising, back in the columbarium, with her new teacher, surrounded by what she loves. It's been twelve years. She might even be good by now.

Anne Elliott is a spoken word artist/ukulelist living in Brooklyn, NY. Her work has appeared in Poetry Nation: The North American Anthology of Fusion Poetry (Vehicule) *and other anthologies. Her blog: http://assbackwords.blogspot.com.*

Centre of Dread

Faye George

Diagnosis

I must be careful to let everyone hug me.
Just when I think no one is left
who has not heard the story:
how I found out my body was unfaithful,
I must tell it again from the beginning.

The children come looking for me
in the house of their childhood,
forgetting I, too, have moved away.
We are all here in a different place
together now, scared and telling jokes.

Tumour

At the centre of dread
a dark mass glistens,
pearl of great price, locked

in the little rib cradle
under the soft layers
next to my heart.

How long it has swelled
in its moist nest
seeding the blood,

no one knows.
Smooth, brooding,
inscrutable pod,

a frigid sun
that sucks me into its orbit,
that clouds the eyes of my friends.

Post Op

I wrote on the release form
that I wanted to keep my kidney
for a paperweight,
but no one paid attention.

They wheeled me into surgery
and cut it out—
a vase with two dark flowers
delivered to pathology—

and told me how lucky I was
to be rid of it,
like a bad kid
that has left home for good.

But the body never gives up its own.
The body mourns—
depression, hormones:
loss is loss.

Surgical Scar

The little pink path that the knife took
slips like the hand of a lover
from waist to breast and gets lost,
like the head of a worm, deep in.

The little pink path that is numb now
where the blood ran when the gloved hand
pressed the cold steel down
and the flesh cracked in a scarlet path

to the trusted thing that shaped in the dark
its terrible wrong, its terrible wrong.

Faye George, a Perugia Press Prize winner, has authored three books of poetry; her latest is Märchenhaft, Like a Fairy Tale. Her poems have appeared in Paris Review, Poetry, and the Poetry Anthology, 1912–2002.

At Thirteen, Asthmatic

John Grey

Our house succumbs to black.
I try to catch the eye of sidewalks,
but the colours, the cloth, the flesh tones,
hurt more than they dazzle.

Our house goes down with
the church spire and the hardware store.
It is lost to night life
like a drowning man a mile from shore.

Some laughter busts through but cuts the ears.
Even a soft kiss can travel this far,
but by the time it gets here,
is dead from the journey.

Our house shrinks to fit inside
my pajama pocket as I struggle upstairs
to my bedroom, wheezing and
grabbing at my chest.

There's a lover out there
who's waiting for me.
For now, she's not winnable.
For now, she is oxygen.

Medicine Pudding

Lumpy, curdled,
you sit on my plate like a swamp.
You're the colour of bile.
One bite and you twist my mouth
in your vise, suck my tongue
like a toothless street woman.

But the doctor says you are perfection,
you know exactly what is bad and kill it.
Why pretend to be food is your motto.
No sweet, no rich, no creamy,
but whom would I rather have when
the enemy attacks—poets or soldiers?

I feel worse, of course, try as you might
to convince me your vile taste
will be my succulent salvation in time.
Cure more wretched than disease.
You enjoy being a metaphor too much,
that's your problem.

First Day Home from the Hospital

I was the first one out on the street
after the rain.
I felt like the air, cool and clean.
Every shop window I passed
was dark and chintzy
compared to my clarity

and feeling of great worth.
I could feel my thoughts
cleansing my body.
I wanted to tell people
my face was the truth,
only there was nobody else
out and about.
The rain stopped, and here I was.
I had timed it just right,
and no one else
had been so fortunate.
The sun poked through the clouds,
like a god I didn't even have
to ask for.
The breeze did its quick
diagnostic flutter
and blew on,
convinced I didn't have
an unhealthy bone in my body.
It could have been Paris or Venice
or the North Pole,
but it was my neighbourhood,
and despite all of the choices
the moment could have made,
it picked me
and glowed with the wisdom
of its selection.

John Grey, an Australian-born poet, playwright, and musician, U.S. resident since the late 1970s, was recently published in Inscape, Halifax Review, *and* South Carolina Review. *His latest book is* What Else Is There? *(Main Street Rag).*

Daughter Cells

Jessica Handler

One morning in July, I sat in a hard plastic chair and let a lab technician strap my left forearm pinch-tight with a rubber tube. After the needle's sting, I turned my gaze away. Watching my body relinquish secrets, I was only beginning to learn that what it kept made me queasy. This blood test took longer than those I had sat through before. On this day, the lab technician filled test tube after test tube with my blood. Only after she snapped the rubber choke from my skin and touched my drowsing arm with icy alcohol did I feel steady enough to direct my sight back to the lab tech. On the counter behind her, half a dozen vials of my blood, viscous as tomato juice, stood upright in the kind of dimpled tray that might hold eggs. Every tube was jammed shut with a blue rubber stopper. On every tube was a sticker with my name on it: "J. Handler/Sibling."

I was nine years old and had come to the lab with my parents and my sisters to try to help piece together the genetic puzzle that had caused my sisters' health to fail. Susie, seven at the time of this blood test, had been diagnosed with leukemia the year before. Sarah, then three, had been born with an immune-system deficiency called Kostmann's syndrome. Her body was unable to produce an adequate amount of neutrophils, a type of white blood cells, and she was susceptible to every germ. Nothing was wrong with me.

Leukemia and Kostmann's syndrome are bone marrow failures. Leukemia is an overabundance of white blood cells, Kostmann's syndrome an almost total absence of them. Lack of white blood cells can be a side effect of chemotherapy (which is itself a treatment for leukemia), but if you are born with it, you have a genetic anomaly. Both parents have to carry the rare gene for Kostmann's syndrome in order for the disease to be present in their child.

Leukemia, too, can be hereditary, or it can be the result of environmental factors. Scientists investigated the "why" of childhood leukemia long before my sister became ill. The studies are endless; one recent study claims nightlights as a culprit, other studies argue against microwave ovens, pesticides, or radon. Another points to exposure to industrial wastes like benzene. Leukemia can develop from a mix of causes, becoming a monster swaying to life when genetic predisposition to the disease meets a troubled natural environment.

Leukemia is common in children: some estimates say nearly three thousand new cases are diagnosed every year in the United States. Kostmann's syndrome is so unusual that, worldwide, it is seen only in about one in two million births. How did two out of three sisters develop hereditary disorders that live at opposite ends of a spectrum? Doctors pronounced us a bizarre coincidence. We were mystified, and so was every doctor we met.

Summer 1969

SHEPHERDED BY OUR PARENTS, Sarah, Susie, and I walked across the blistering black tarmac at Atlanta's airport and up rollaway stairs into the plane. The five of us flew to Durham, North Carolina, for a series of blood tests that might or might not reveal where our reverse miracle had come from.

We were sophisticated kids, accustomed to flying and the accompanying marvel of sitting down to breakfast in one city and to lunch in another. We flew to New York every winter to visit aunts and uncles and cousins and to trek through museums and giant department stores. When we were done, we ate with chopsticks in Chinatown. In the summer, we flew to Pennsylvania and to Massachusetts to stay with our grandparents. A two-day trip to Duke University was no more to us than another visit to another hospital. We were prepared to fulfill our responsibility to more doctors—interchangeable with the ones at home—and to our parents before we got to play in the motel pool or dress up to go out for dinner at a steakhouse. We were polite. We presented our left arms, sleeves rolled up, for the needle. We gently flicked our fingers against the soft insides of our elbows to raise the big vein there, showing off just a little bit for the lab tech. Our frankness made her stare. We answered questions; how old each of was, how we were feeling, what was the name of Sarah's stuffed bear.

Intending to be helpful, I confided in Dr. B., a blonde woman who appeared no older than the nursing student who babysat us at home. "I'm the well sibling," I announced as I shook her hand. I noticed that she chose not to write this insight on her clipboard. After each of us relinquished vial after vial of blood and my parents completed pages of paperwork, we left the lab. Mom carried Sarah, Dad walked just ahead with a file under his arm, Susie and I brought up the rear. Susie fainted while we waited for the elevator. When she crumpled to the linoleum, my parents' calm shattered: Mom screamed, Dad swore, a male nurse in white came running. I was afraid. As sick as I knew Susie and Sarah were, any physical evidence of their fallibility had up until then been confined to the days when they were patients in a hospital. No one ever fainted or threw up or had a nosebleed in street clothes. I have never since seen a child collapse.

We did not go as a family for more tests after that single day. There was nothing anyone could tell us about why death sat so close by my sisters, and nothing anyone could do to shoo death away. There were no answers to the question of why two diseases struck my family like rogue lightning out of a clear sky, hitting my sisters and bypassing me. Genetics is a good guess. So is bad luck.

Fall 1975

I NEARLY DRIED UP and died of boredom on the subject of genetics in my Grade 10 biology class. Dissecting leathery cats and frogs unnerved me. Mendel and his peas blossomed into tedium. Our teacher's lectures on *Drosophila*—fruit flies—generated snarky remarks among the bored kids at the back table. We cracked ourselves up with puns like "be fruit fly and multiple," and learned nothing about this first draft of genetic mapping. "Ontogeny recapitulates phylogeny" stayed with me only because of its catchy, bumpety-bump rhythm. The phrase means that every embryo's development mirrors the entire evolutionary process;

eons of practised, mindless change whiz through the earliest moments of every organism like a time-lapse film. Having been studied some myself, I was secretly disappointed that I was not able to relate to the *Drosophila*.

Open my veins and coax information out. Find the answer to my parents' anguish and tell me if I will face the same. Isolate the random error in our genetic code as if you were fishing macaroni letters from a bowl of alphabet soup. Because I knew early on that a lab technician was looking for mutations in my family's cells, I believed that at our most primitive level, my family was different from others. If we had a mutation then we would be freaks. Almost immediately, I became fascinated by stories about Chang and Eng, twins conjoined by a band of flesh at their chests, or with tales of General Tom Thumb and his bride Lavinia Warren. Leafing through my parents' book of Diane Arbus photographs, I happened on a portrait of lunkish and tragic Eddie Carmel, who at a purported nine feet tall, towered over his stunned parents. I opened the book to "Jewish Giant in the Bronx" over and over again, wondering how Eddie could sleep comfortably in bed and if his back ached from bending so low to walk through doorways.

My mother tells me now that she and my father heard the whispers and felt the stares when they walked the halls of children's hospitals. Other parents were always empathic as they escaped their child's room for a blessedly vacant moment in the cafeteria or the gift shop. These parents were also relieved once they had made the obvious comparisons. They might have one child vomiting from chemotherapy, sleeping through post-op recovery, or dying, but in Susie and Sarah, my parents had two.

In elementary school I rescued Susie's stiff wig from the red clay playground dirt. A Grade 7 bully had torn the wig from her bald head and flung it, horrified, onto the dodge-ball court. Of course I rushed to save the hair, returning it like a furry pet to my stunned little sister. Of course we were the only children on the playground who knew how to place the hair on her naked head. Susie centred it like a hat, then mashed down hard, pressing a new strip of plastic tape into place against her skull.

Winter 1990

BEING THE WELL SIBLING meant agreeing instantly to be the donor for Sarah's bone-marrow transplant. This was no guaranteed cure, but any source of rest for the weary. Envisioning exposing my hip or sternum to a needle to relinquish a quart of marrow made my knees go weak. The flesh between my shoulder blades crawled. Of course I would spend six months in a hospital for you. In one room I would grow pale and weak before my certain rebound. In the next, you would pink up, nourished from the meat inside my bones.

The idea was that my white blood cells might grow in Sarah's body and provide her immune system with a new start. Statistically, siblings—allogeneic donors—are the closest match.

"This is going to be harder on you than it is on me," Sarah said. We were talking on the telephone, me at the southern end of the Eastern Seaboard, she at the northern. Each of us was grown, or nearly so. I demurred and made comforting words, thinking I could deflect her fear. "I can manage a hospital stay," I said, all bravado. Anxious to feel nothing, I talked but didn't listen. I could never be her or understand what it meant to live her life. Her words bounced off me with a pinging sound. She was hail, I was a tin roof.

"That's not what I mean," Sarah said. Her voice was tight, testy. As if she were talking to a lost child, as if she were the big sister and I the small one, she went on. "When I die. You know that's what I mean." You won't die, I thought. You can't.

OUR FAMILY'S INSCRUTABLE GENETICS re-emerged with the results of my preliminary blood test. I was not a donor match for Sarah. Nor were our parents, aunts, uncles, cousins, or friends. Susie might have been a match, but she was dead.

Sarah and I talked around our disappointment, treading gently around the holes opening in our hearts. Her death was closer than ever, and we knew it. Instead, we laughed hard when we spoke about her new car, our mother's birthday, my boyfriend troubles.

From the outside, you couldn't tell that ours was a family with a genetic mutation. I am tall. I am big-boned and have dark hair. I look like what I am: a genetic combination of my parents. Had Susie lived longer than the age of eight, she would have been a tallish woman like I am. Her hair was dark and wavy, like mine. In photographs of the two of us together, I see now that her grin was wider than mine, a characteristic of personality rather than science. All of us sisters inherited our parents' jutting jaw. We had in common the same swimmer's shoulders and broad rib cages. When she did die at the age of twenty-seven, Sarah was five feet tall, although I can hear her insisting that she was five feet one. She was also honey-blonde. Her hair colour was a genetic throwback some unknown number of generations. No one I can think of in our family is fair, but then again, the first cases of Kostmann's syndrome have been traced to Sweden. Most Swedes are blonde. Sweden is proximate to Russia, Poland, and Lithuania, where my grandparents, their parents, and members of generations rolling back in time were born. Genes have long memories.

In the sixteenth century, French surgeon Ambroise Paré addressed the titillation factor that attends the realities of being born different. In his *Monstres et Prodiges* he attributes thirteen causes of deformity and illness (thirteen being the timeless number for the superstitious). One reason was the disruptive presence of "demons and devils." Another cause, Paré claimed, was the pregnant woman's sitting in an "unbecoming manner," crossing her legs or pulling her knees under her chin. He was prescient in his suggestion of a ninth possible origin. That, he wrote, was "heredity and accidental illness."

Every time a cell divides, two identical new cells are made. These are daughter cells. When they divide again, you have two more daughter cells. Errors can occur. Not all genes from the original cell may make it into the daughter cell. Sometimes more than one copy of a chromosome develops in a daughter cell, diverting normal development. Most of us live lucky lives, the probability of our staying reasonably healthy asserted early in our genes. Our children should be born healthy, but sometimes they arrive ill-equipped, unable to dodge their fate. I am insensible of the potential for cruelty within my cells.

Spring 1998

MY HUSBAND AND I sat holding hands in an overheated medical centre conference room. We had come for genetic counselling. We had given blood, and now we had to listen to a dark-haired woman in a lab coat chirp statistics about mutations, defects, and the rate of healthy pregnancies for women in their forties. As she flipped laminated pages on a chart, my thoughts wandered to Mendel's peas. In my mind, the phrase changed—mutated—to "Mengele's peas." On the plastic cards in front of us, blown-up photographs of someone else's genes, used as lecture aids, appeared to wind around themselves like tapeworms.

Having seen up close the losses I could experience as a mother, I wanted to know for certain that I would not meet my family's troubles again. Prove that to me, I want to say. Show me which of my parent's genes met and created mutations, or why my sister's genes altered in the womb. Show me which genes of mine, if any, are poised to communicate more bad news.

No one can guarantee me this peace of mind. Susie and Sarah would tell you that they were more than their illnesses. They were smart, beautiful girls. They had outrageous senses of humour. Susie once pestered our mother at a grocery store meat department until she surrendered and handed over some change for a pair of disembodied chicken feet.

"Mom, please," Susie pleaded. Pushing her nose against the curved glass case, she couldn't take her eyes away from the scaly, grey-clawed feet on ice. Mom took her wallet from her purse to pay the man, and Susie held her hand up for the white paper package. At kindergarten the next day, Susie used the splayed yellow feet as stamps in a dish of tempera paint. On her strip of paper (the other kids used raw potatoes cut in half to imprint flower shapes and smiles and trapezoids), ghost chickens marched across a paper road.

When Sarah was in junior high school, she signed notes "love and other indoor sports." She called me in my college dorm to tell me her first dirty joke. "What do you call a mushroom that's long and hard?" she giggled. "A fungi to be with."

We were three sisters, we were not freaks.

Wrestling with how our genetic makeup defined our lives has given me another taste of my childhood alphabet soup. I have learned that DNA is made of four chemical compounds; adenine, guanine, cytosine, and thymine. Called A, G, C, and T, they are the four-letter alphabet floating in everyone's bowl. I know enough now about the subject I loathed in high school to assign a basic concept to words like *chromosome* and *allogeneic*. That's enough for me.

When I look at photographs of Sarah and Susie and me, or read our aging diary entries and birthday cards and letters written in loopy girl-script, I see the truest things I need to know about the girls we were.

When the lightning that struck two out of three little girls can be named and the place where it came to rest in their bodies can be located, then a new caring person in a lab coat can pick up where an earlier one left off, and show me the scorched place inside my own body.

Jessica Handler's first book is Invisible Sisters: A Memoir. *She received Special Mention for a 2008 Pushcart Prize and the 2009 Peter Taylor Nonfiction Fellowship at the Kenyon Review Writers Workshop.*

BSE

Alison Hauch

Jillian liked the shower hot. It was best when it fogged up the mirrors and made the towels damp. Since the bathroom fan had been broken before they moved into the house seven years earlier, it never took long before she could see the walls start to sweat. It made the paint crack and peel and her husband was forever asking her to open the window and let the heat out. And while she understood the need to save the walls from collapsing like candy floss, usually she forgot. It wasn't on purpose; it was just the last thing on her mind when she turned the handle and walked out the door.

On the rare occasion she remembered to open the window, she always wondered how it looked from the outside with billows of steam puffing out. It was as if her house had held its breath and finally decided to exhale in relief. That thought amused her and she sometimes watched the steam curl away, but to be perfectly truthful, most of the time she forgot to open the window at all. It was sort of the same way her husband forgot about his plans to fix the fan every summer. It was amazing, she thought, as she popped the clear plastic lid off her new, disposable pink-as-bubblegum razor—like shaving was somehow a treat to be savoured—that someone could forget to do something for seven years. After all, it only takes nine months to make an entire baby. It only takes a year to get a divorce. It only takes six weeks to die after the doctors finally figure out that it's cancer. Seven years to fix a fan seemed a bit disproportionate and trivial at the same time, sort of like taking a limousine out to buy garbage bags or sewing sequins on a dishcloth. It wasn't as though there were never any reminders, but it somehow escaped both of them every time they left their tiny turquoise bathroom with the claw-foot tub.

And seven years was a long time to live with just one bathroom anyway, she decided as she shrugged out of her old, white bathrobe, especially now that her twin daughters wanted to bathe separately, the joy of communal cleaning waning as the parameters of the tub became too small to share. Seven years was a long time to put up with the shower curtain sticking to her legs as she tried to shave, balanced on one slippery foot, right hand carving out tracks of hairless skin as the left hand swatted away wet vinyl that seemed to be attracted to her skin the way mustard was attracted to white shorts. And seven years was a long time to repeat the monthly five-step ritual in this tiny, airless, steamy space. Seven years times twelve months made eighty-four rituals. Eighty-four rituals times five steps made four hundred and twenty steps. She had done the ritual eighty-four times. She had taken four hundred and twenty steps. And each time she held her breath, made sure her hands were warm enough and slippery enough and wished that she were seven minutes away into the future and not stuck here with seven minutes left to go.

Step One: Strip to the waist. Stand in front of the mirror with your hands on your hips. Take a good, hard look at yourself. Remember to breathe. Are your breasts their usual size, shape, and colour? Are both your nipples "outies," not "innies"? No sinister dimples? No icky rashes? No odd pimples? No sneaky puckers? No unsightly bulges?

Proceed.

Jillian had loved being a girl. She loved being a woman even more. Not for one moment in her life did she ever wish to be anything other than what she was, which was female from her inside out. But sometimes—once a month, her time of the month, when she got her monthly bill—she was afraid of herself. She didn't like how strange it felt to be afraid of the skin she wore every day. It seemed wrong to fear the body that had so far proven smart enough to grow up and out in all the right directions, organized enough to oversee the production of two tiny humans, nurturing enough to handle all her bad decisions and forgiving enough to deal with her regular need for chocolate and French bread.

Step Two: Now raise your arms and look for the same things. See if a youthful lift changes the landscape. Try not to yearn for the days when the girls sat up this high all on their own. Confused? Forgotten your clues? Refer back to Step One. And keep breathing.

Proceed.

Because much as she loved being female, two of the most tangible symbols of womanhood—her tits, her ta-tas, her hooters, her jugs, her knockers, her rack, her boobs, her bazooms, her breasts—went from being her best friends, the kind of friends she could count on to fill her up and fill her out just right, to being her biggest foes, the kind that filled her with anxiety. And all the silly, fluffy, bunny names in the world could not disguise the fact that while they seemed soft and gentle, they could easily turn on her, like a stinky cheese left a few days too long.

It was the only love-hate relationship she had ever really had.

She loved the way they looked in her white tank top, but she hated the way her hormones made them hot and heavy. She loved how they balanced out the curve of her hips and matched the number of her legs, but she hated how they stole the attention she sometimes needed to give the other sum of her parts. She loved the way they fed two lives well enough to navigate them through their first few years, but she hated the way they collected cells and scrunched them into cysts and bumps and lumps—scary, undefined bubbles under translucent skin—like swamp gas beneath the bog of her bra.

Step Three: Gently squeeze each nipple between your pointer finger and your thumb. Ignore any vaguely porn star-ish sensations. Remember to breathe. Check for any discharge. Is it milky? Is it bloody? Is it yellowy or stinky or any of the other seven dwarves?

Proceed.

As the time got closer each month, the time when she had to pick her way through the maze of her own flesh seeking out any tiny anomaly (trying to remember last month's trek and wishing she had drawn a map) she worried and wondered. Jillian stewed in a juice full of memories of dead mothers and staggering statistics, of pink ribbons and health advisories, and she watched her girls and hoped she would find her way out successfully again this month so that the word *mama* didn't become part of a dead language to them, the way the word *grandma* had.

Step Four: This is the biggie. Pay attention. Don't get lost. Lie down and cop a feel. Pretend it is a prelude to sex, not cysts. Feel your breasts with your opposite hands. Use the pads of your first few fingers. Make sure you feel from stem to stern, port to starboard, cleavage to shoulder blade. Start at your nipple and move your hands in larger and larger circles until you've spiralled out to the edge. Then give the vertical plane a whirl. Go in rows, as if you are painting a wall. Start pressing softly and then repeat, pressing harder. Sorry to those of you who are sensitive. But press on you must. Stop holding your breath. What should your breasts feel like? Excellent question. They could feel like lumpy oatmeal or a rubbery ball. Parts of your breast might feel like a sea sponge or the white of a slightly cooked egg. Know your breasts. Learn your breasts. Love your breasts. Take stock of your breasts. Any lumps? Any thick bits? Any spots that don't move when stuck between a rib and a hard place?

Proceed.

Jillian loved the elation she felt when she discovered her mammary intelligence had managed to keep the status quo for another twenty-eight days. But she hated it that the elation came not from any gain, but from merely staying the same. There was never any chance for improvement in this game. It was maintain or decline. Just once she would like some way to gauge whether the result was actually healthier, happier, safer. Wouldn't it be great to know that she had done some magical thing to actually come out even better than the time before? She had always liked going forward. Staying still made her anxious, and moving backwards was terrifying. But in this situation there was no way to move ahead. And so she had to accept that no news is good news.

Step Five: It's time to mix the wet and dry ingredients together. You need to feel your breasts while standing or sitting. Now the shower comes in handy. It's easiest to do your pushing and prodding when you are wet and slippery—as is true of so many things.

Remember what you did in Step Four. Lube up your hands and get to it. Any surprises? Any shocking change of events? Come on now; you're not breathing.

Proceed.

But what she hated the most, what she struggled with more than anything else was the time she wasted beforehand—a week of mental preparation the way a sprinter visualizes a race. She resented the way the impending ritual weighed on all her joys and lightness, deflating them like dropping stones on soap bubbles. It didn't matter how many voices told her to put it out of her mind, to ignore it until the time came, to put it in a box to take out once each moon; she could never escape that presence in the back of her mind, squatting like a turnip, growing and growing until its monthly harvest. Like a woman's cycle, she lathered, rinsed, and repeated, elation to fear, fear to elation, always hoping that she wouldn't find the thing that makes elation impossible, but secretly worrying that she would. And she hoped for the moments after the ritual to be happy ones, though she thought some might say shaving and washing her hair and cleaning between her toes was anti-climatic by comparison. She disagreed. Those tasks were like the victory lap after pushing her chest through the tape at the finish line; she could see it coming closer and closer as she explored further and further with her fingertips. Those mundane chores were her cool down, her chance to work out the lactic acid that had built up in her brain from the tension of anticipation. She cherished and hoped for that pause at the top of the five long steps and sometimes just let the hot spray hit her face as she cupped her breasts and celebrated another month.

Conclusion: Now that the exam is completed, take note of anything troublesome you saw or felt during Steps One through Five. No trouble spots? Go to Subsection A: get on with your life for the next month. However, if anything is out of place, or you have found something new in place, go immediately to Subsection B: your doctor. They have all manner of devices with which to take a clearer picture of your little gatherings. Try the impossible task of not dwelling on it until you get your results. It might take awhile, so don't hold your breath. Afraid? Understandable, but don't be such a fibroid. It might be nothing.

Proceed.

She pressed the shower button down with her right foot and turned off the water. She wrung out her hair and wrapped it in a pink towel, turban style. She stepped out, dried herself off, and put her old white robe back on. She ran a hand across the foggy mirror—she would have scolded her kids for doing that—looked at herself a moment, and opened the bathroom door. She took two steps out, then turned, came back in, leaned across the tub, pulled the shower curtain out of her way and pushed the window open. No more reason to hold her breath, she and her house exhaled softly together.

Alison is a secondary school dance teacher and mother of two girls. She enjoys spending her free time dancing, reading, and writing. She lost both her mother and her mother-in-law to cancer.

Things Taken

Isabel Hoskins

It was October, the thick middle of autumn, when I had my last period. I remember that I bled onto newly washed sheets. I remember eating pears: green and brown and rusted red, juicy in their perfect ripeness. I remember the headache that started at the base of my spine and twisted its knotted fingers around the right side of my skull, boring into my temple and eye socket. I remember my last period because medical arrangements were made around it, and because while I bled that October, I was very afraid.

I had just returned from my midwife's office where, during my yearly exam, she said she could feel something large and abnormal on my ovary. She told me I needed to make an appointment for an internal ultrasound, that I should get in as soon as possible, but that the test could not be done during my period. I remember sitting at the dining room table, determining where I was in my cycle. The boxes on the calendar, each one with their inked number, said I would begin bleeding in only three days. My appointment was scheduled for that very evening.

Then, for three days I waited for the results of the ultrasound and waited for my last period, which I did not know would be my last. My family history felt like poisoned soil, infecting the tree that bore our names on branches. So I worried I about things like cancer: uterine, cervical, and ovarian. I told myself not to worry because I was young, only thirty. I did what they tell you not to do and researched on the Internet, typing in my symptoms and reading the results with panic. I passed time at home watching episodes of *House* on DVD, as if in viewing each rare and strange disease I would become immune to it. I played hours of mah-jong on the computer. I told myself that if I could win just one game before the results came, the news would be good.

My last period started the day we heard from my midwife, and she told me that the ultrasound revealed there was a mass on each ovary and I needed to see a gynecologist in her practice. My husband and I drove to Dr. Saleh's office an hour later. I was bleeding with my period as we sat in the waiting room, and I played solitaire on Todd's Palm Pilot. I won a game as we sat waiting in the exam room and I told Todd it was a good omen. Not a mah-jong win, but still, it meant something.

Dr. Saleh came in the room and introduced himself. I remember the intoxicating smell of his cologne: pine, cedar, musk, black pepper. He looked at my charts, my results, my body. He said that I had what appeared to be two large cysts, one on each ovary. He said that his opinion was that I should have surgery to remove them as soon as possible, as they were large, the size of oranges and grapefruit, and would likely continue to grow. He said that cysts are benign, but that they can take on a life of their own and sometimes when they remove them, the cysts have hair and teeth growing on them. He said that we should not be worried, that it was quite common to have ovarian cysts, that he was not thinking tumours or cancer and we should not be either. He said he wanted to give me an internal vaginal exam. I told him I was having my period now. He said this was fine, that he was only feeling for the location and size of the cysts. I remember my last period because when he removed his hand from my vagina, the glove was covered in my red menstrual blood and he tried to be discreet while he pulled it off and threw it in the toxic waste bin.

I bled for my normal ten days and during this time I waited for surgery. I remember sitting at my friend's house, and she asked me if I was scared or worried. I told her that, strangely, I was not. I felt like everything would be fine.

"I'm willing to be surprised," I said.

My last period ended. The bright red blood turned to soft pink and then it was done. The box of tampons went back in the linen closet alongside towels and cotton balls and toilet cleaner. Three days later I was at the hospital for surgery. As they wheeled me into the operating room the anesthesiologist asked me if I wanted a little shot of a relaxant, to soften things around the edges before they officially put me under. I said yes. And then I was out and I don't remember what happened because I had fallen into the unconscious, abducted into darkness, the last memory I have, Dr. Saleh leaning over my bed and smelling so good I could have crawled up and rested in the crook of his neck.

I have no memory of the next eight hours. I have been told that this is what happened. Dr. Saleh began the surgery laparoscopically and once inside he discovered a tumour. They slit my skin apart, a horizontal incision just above my pubic bone. An oncologist was called in for a consult. A piece of the tumour was removed, frozen, and sent for immediate biopsy. It came back malignant. While I was still unconscious and on the operating table, the doctors went out to the waiting room where my husband had been sitting alone in fear, wondering why what was supposed to take two to three hours had now surpassed five. They told him what they had found. He gave them permission to perform a full hysterectomy. They removed uterus, tubes, and ovaries, along with samples from other organs and tissue so they could all be sent to pathology to see if cancer had spread. Successfully emptied, they then sewed my skin back together and when I woke later, in the same room I had been in before they wheeled me into surgery, I looked at the clock on the wall. When it said seven o'clock, hours past when it should have been, I knew something had gone wrong.

Though this is what happened to me, it still feels not mine own. I was not conscious, and in the shroud of anesthesia I had no voice or choice. There was not even dreaming. It remains lost time in which, transported to the realm of the unconscious, events unfolded that would change my life. When they cut into my skin and with sterile surgical instruments removed organs and cysts and tumour, they cut open a wound in the ground and, like Persephone abducted into the Underworld by Hades, I slipped underneath.

In the days following, Dr. Saleh and the oncologist came to see me at frequent intervals, telling the same story again and again. I was thirty, so young to have had ovarian cancer. I was amazingly lucky to have had it found in the earliest of stages. I was not to worry because, though we were still waiting for the rest of the results to make sure it had not spread, they found everything so soon and I was so young.

People came to sit with me in the hospital and they said they were sorry and that I was brave. My mom flew out to take care of things at home. My midwife, who had been with me for the birth of my son, cried when she came to see me. The nurses warned me it would take a long time to recover, longer than the six weeks for my body to heal. The oncologist reminded me every time she stopped in my room how lucky I was, how remarkable really it was that I figured this out when I did. My husband reminded me, himself, again and again, "We were not planning on having any more kids anyway."

The pathology results returned and, except for the tumour and right ovary, they were all negative. A week later I went to see the oncologist and she told me I had been diagnosed with stage 1C ovarian cancer and that I required no further cancer treatments such as radiation or chemotherapy, as all cancer was successfully removed during surgery. She told me I would need to take tumour marker tests every six months for the next several years. She told me I would probably experience depression.

AND THEN MY MOM returned home. And then Todd went back to work. And then it was Halloween and I was well enough to walk slowly through the street with my toddler while he went trick-or-treating, the tail of his furry Tigger costume trailing behind. And then I went for the two-week post-surgical checkup with Dr. Saleh. Cancer free. Lucky. The incision healing well, quickly, faster than expected. And then the ground closed over me, from that place where I descended, and the grass grew over what had been a gaping wound and it was still, as if nothing ever happened.

I recovered, regained strength, and resumed normal responsibilities. I had not planned on having more children anyway. I was fortunate. I had known worse things than the loss of my reproductive organs. I was grateful for my life, my husband, my health, my son. I was young, only thirty, and my body could bounce back. If it were not for my absent menstrual cycle, I could pretend everything was normal.

I tried to make the most of things and went shopping for all new underwear, pretty delicate things that would never be stained with blood because I miscalculated the beginning of period or went out without bringing an extra tampon. That was it then. My consolation for losing my uterus and estrogen, for being cut open and stripped of organs, was twelve new pairs of panties. The absurdity slapped me and I felt a stinging burn through my body. Back home, looking through my purchases, I started crying. I did not stop. In the thicket of the unconscious and unspoken, in my fears and feelings that oozed and wormed their way into my dreams, in the images that arose from the part of me still locked against my will in that place to which I had descended, I began to grieve.

It was in the terrain of my flesh, with its scar ripping across my lower abdomen, with its absence of estrogen and progesterone, with its memory, that I found the way to mourn and tell my story. At times the grief felt like an emptiness, a void, barren as my removed womb. Where I once felt fertile creativity, there was vacancy. Absence itself came to take up space. My body began to dry out. I watched my hair change texture and turn to frizz, refusing to hold soft curls. My skin revealed its parched patches, flaking as if they had seen the scorch of desert heat. I found myself unable to wear contact lenses because even my eyes had lost their slippery wetness. Sometimes in the arid starkness of loss it felt as if nothing could grow on such a desolate land. My body taught me how to grieve.

It has been a year since my last period. I am still grieving. I grieve what I have lost and what has been given: the innocence of believing that youth equals health, the baffling realization I had cancer and it was both discovered and eradicated all while unconscious, the absence of my reproductive organs and the hormones that affect more than I had imagined, the ability to have a choice in whether or not I would have another child birthed from my body, the doctor visits that clutter my calendar, that vulnerability of having my insides touched and parts of me taken. And this: I miss my period.

It happened so suddenly, with no warning of its departure, and I miss my periods. I miss bleeding once a month. I miss the movement of feelings, the undulation of energy and creativity and how, though always fluctuating, it followed a rhythm, predictable and cyclical and intimate.

My periods have left me. Weeks pass, months pass, seasons shape shift, and I no longer know this in my body as I once did. For eighteen years menstruation has been the way I tell time, the circling of ovulation and emptying. It is more to me than just a physiological process of egg descending down the tube, of the lining on the uterus growing thick and webbed, ready to sustain new life, of the shedding of blood that has been considered to be both sacred and unclean. For me, having my period was how my body spoke to me and how I began listening. The entire life cycle was found with my own flesh, the beginning and ending and beginning again. I miss my periods, the shedding of blood like snakes slithering out of their skin.

Time passes. I move on, but not as I once was. In the shadow of fecundity is that which destroys and takes from us in its descent, returning us to the womb so we might begin again. Even without my periods a life cycle remains in me. As Persephone heralding the first stirrings of spring, I walk again upon the earth. The Underworld does not leave me but comes with me, rooted in my body as I grieve its wounds. I feel the physical manifestations of menopause and the emotional aftermath of being cut open, with its grief and anger and gratitude for saving me, and I watch myself fuse back together, the way my skin did as it healed from its surgical wound.

It is October once again and there are pumpkins and squash and the first pomegranates of the season with the thick, husk-like skin puckered up at the top like a kiss, the lumpy roundness, the hidden nest of seeds. I buy one and bring it home, slicing through the middle where it then falls into two halves and a tiny stream of juice drips onto the counter. Inside is a mine of jewel-toned seeds, each one a morsel of tart sweetness, beginning with a delicate crunch and softening into liquid centre. There is no real fleshy meat. The seeds are the meat, the prize, the delicacy, the red gift. And there are so many, too many to count, and they remind me of my lost eggs from my lost ovaries that were once inside my body and now are no longer. I pull the seeds out with my fingers, disentangling them from the webbed centre. They feel like pearls, smooth, but if you put them in between your teeth, you can feel their gritty beginnings. I eat the seed, swallow it whole.

Isabel Hoskins is a writer and licensed doula. Currently a student at Goddard College, she is studying the mythological, medical, and personal history of the womb. She lives in Chicago, Illinois, with her husband and son.

Pain Scale

Paul Hostovsky

I'm waiting for my doctor in this little room,
all alone with my body and nothing to read
except for the anatomy chart and the Lipitor ad,
and tacked to the wall near the blood pressure cuff
this other small piece of paper with six
progressively withering smiley faces
numbered zero to five. How do I know it's a pain scale
for the non-verbal, or the non-English-speaking,
or maybe the deaf? It's gotten my attention
as only pain can. I imagine my doctor asking,
"How much does it hurt?" then pointing to each
corroding happy face in turn with a trembling
index. The first face boasts a smile a hundred
and eighty degrees wide, labelled zero for zero pain.
The last face is wringing tears from the scrunched up
lines that make up its face, labelled five for crushing
pain. And the faces in between, one through four,
might be mild, annoying, pounding, wrenching
pain. That is if there were words for what is all
vowels anyway. I mean, what can you say about pain
when ouch says it all; when words at their best
are merely true—or merely due, like the blessing
after achoo; when the complete works of Shakespeare
couldn't budge one kidney stone, nor all the Bibles
in all the hotel rooms piled on top of each other reach
the big toe of the suicide hanging in 14B . . . I mean
you'd think we'd have figured it out by now, what to do
with all the pain, what to make of it, this natural
resource everywhere abundantly fallow, in every

corner of the world, every corner of the body. You'd think
by now we'd have invented a formula for converting it
into energy or food, or cancelling it out completely,
dividing it by itself or the farthest star, or else some
denominator we have yet to imagine. But no, when it comes
to pain, we're still in kindergarten. When it comes,
we can only hunch over it, try to draw from memory
the irretrievable face of happiness. The language
of pain is wind in a field, it's wind howling past a useless
tongue, past lips and teeth like disused rails and ties
abandoned in a field, where once the excellent trains ran
all day and into the night, the well-timed, smart arrivals.

Paul Hostovsky's poems have won a Pushcart Prize, the Muriel Craft Bailey Award from the Comstock Review, and chapbook contests from Grayson Books, Riverstone Press, and the Frank Cat Press. Visit his website: www.paulhostovsky.com.

Seeing the Heart

Catherine Jagoe

The great-grandmother from Mexico
lies meekly on the gurney
fumbles at her hair with her soft hands
before they immobilize
her arms, stick metal-nippled
patches to her chest, infuse
her with blood thinner,
shave her pubis, swab
her white thigh brown with iodine
lay out the ceremonial green
cloths for the square hole of flesh
scrub their hands and arms up to the elbows
unpeel sealed gloves, don
plastic goggles and lead aprons
and feed their tubes and dyes
snaking through her groin
towards the chambers of her heart.
The great white eye above her
descends, turns, retracts, pores repeatedly
over her chest.
Clicks and whirrs.
"Look at the screen!" they tell her.
"You can see the blockage clearly!"
Snakeroot. Clematis climbs, winds
tendrils, knots, blooms.
Darkness bleeds like smoke from a branch.
It is not blood, they reassure her, only dye.
The blockage is the blank space in the vine.
They send expandable balloons

to cross the space, while in a monotone
she blesses them, blesses them
continually, barely pausing for breath:
the doctors, the technicians,
the nurses, the stretcher-wheeling man.
Rains blessings on them all
and all their families.
When it is done and they ask,
"Were you afraid?" she says, "No,
porque soy la hija de un rey."
I am the daughter of a king.
And then, both proud and casual:
"His name is Jesus Christ."

Catherine Jagoe is a writer, translator, and medical interpreter in Madison, Wisconsin. Her poetry has been featured on National Public Radio and the Poetry Daily website in the United States.

Matter and Energy

Lorie Kolak

Because of his heart condition, Alan feared he would die in bed and the woman with him that night would scream under the burden of his body. He was twenty-two years old and the doctors predicted he wouldn't pass his thirtieth birthday. Since Alan hadn't time to lose, he planned to spend his remaining days in search of the beautiful and the soft. His great consolation was women: blonde and brunette and raven-haired women, public relations professionals with blown-dry hair and tailored suits, college girls with loud laughs who gave him dirty nicknames. He was a man of the finger and of the palm. He slowed down when most men rushed (or so he was told), and he stared at women with an intensity that made them afraid to ask about love. As his skin was pale, his freckles girlish, his files organized, Alan was glad to tell stories of his conquests to the men at the accounting firm where he worked. He found solace in concentrating on the pleasures of a woman's body when he was so pained by his own.

ALAN DIDN'T BRING A DATE to the wedding where he met Bettina, and she, too, had come alone. He watched her arrange the neck of her black dress, tugging it down across her breasts. She pushed her brown hair behind her ears, frowned, and glanced sideways. Alan watched the neck of the ill-fitting dress rise up again, as if pulled by the force of her awkwardness.

"Are you on the bride's side or the groom's?" Alan asked, sitting down at her table.

"I'm on her side," she said, "but he's already won."

"You don't like him."

"He's making her negotiate with him to keep her job."

"What's her job?" he asked.

"Secretary."

"His?"

"He thinks marriage should change her work status," Bettina continued.

"Do you think she deserves a raise?"

Bettina glared at him.

"I think you deserve one," Alan said.

While the bride and groom were cutting the cake, Alan and Bettina were in a coat closet. Bettina gripped the dowel rod above her head and did not moan or whisper his name or do the things women do. Even at the end, she was silent and so was he. Only when he looked at her face, flushed, her eyebrows raised, her mouth open, could he tell that she was responding. When it was over, she pulled up her nylons, pulled down her black dress, and pushed the coats back.

"Thanks," she said and left.

When Alan returned to the wedding, he watched Bettina talk to the bartender about imported vodkas. She ignored Alan, and this surprised him, because after his other sexual encounters, women wanted to linger in bed and name their children. He tapped Bettina on the shoulder and asked her to dance. She put her drink down and walked to the dance floor.

"Did you like that?" Alan asked, pushing himself up against her.

She shrugged. "You want a ribbon?"

"I want an acknowledgment."

"We had sex."

"We had great sex," Alan said. "Can I take you to dinner?"

WHEN ALAN ASKED BETTINA about herself, she responded in short answers, pushing fries through ketchup, watching the Chicago Bears on a sports bar television, smoking cigarettes on the stoop of her bungalow in a northern suburb of the city. He discovered she was the daughter of a pastor and a nurse. Saturdays, she went to garage sales in other suburbs and small towns all the way to Wisconsin. She bought knick-knacks, church coffee mugs, and sweaters she'd never wear. Alan came to believe the ill-fitting black dress was pulled off a folding table in a driveway. She was eight years older than him and left a man she called "The Architect" at the altar. Her voice dropped to a whisper when she spoke about him.

"Why did you leave him?" Alan asked.

"I wanted to keep him in anticipation," Bettina said. "He never saw it coming. Some architect."

She had a PhD in physics that she used in a regional science laboratory.

"How?"

"Testing."

"Testing what?"

Bettina smiled. "Matter and energy."

Only when Alan told Bettina about his condition, the disease called IHSS, which caused a toughening of the heart's walls, did Bettina ask questions about him. She asked about the rate of his deterioration, the medicine he took, the possible complications of a heart transplant, which hospitals specialized in his illness, and how he felt about planning for the future knowing that he was not predicted to live far into adulthood. He sensed that she was researching what he told her. She insisted on going to a doctor's appointment with him after he passed out while walking to the grocery store. After a series of appointments, his doctor implanted a pacemaker.

"When I was a kid, I had a talking stuffed rabbit," Bettina whispered one night when they lay in bed. She put her hand over the boxy protuberance on his chest and lightly stroked his skin. "It required batteries and I had to pull back a layer of cloth to reach the connections."

He drew her to him and kissed her mouth. Bettina asked for little commitment from him, and in response he wanted to commit everything to her. This was a feeling he'd never known, and he hesitated to call it love, but it brought him great comfort and made him think of his illness differently. He didn't want her to miss him when he was gone. Bettina introduced Alan to a couple who lived next door to her bungalow. On weeknights, with the couple's newborn twins asleep on the rug, they played spades. Bettina insisted on being on a separate team from Alan because she loved telling him which cards he held in his hand, and she always guessed correctly.

AFTER THREE MORE FAINTING SPELLS, Alan tried to negotiate working from home with his boss, but the accounting firm was inflexible. The men at the firm touched his shoulder in sympathy and waited to hear more conquest stories. When he had nothing to offer, they assumed his silence was because of his illness, not because he had fallen in love. He continued working until Bettina proposed to him when they were attending a neighbourhood garage sale. She drove to each house so Alan would not have to walk more than the length of a driveway.

"I was thinking I could marry you," she said, digging through a box of hardback novels.

"I wouldn't have guessed you're the marrying kind," he said.

"You're in trouble."

"I am," Alan said. He pulled out an iron tool from a wooden crate.

"Fifty dollars," a man sitting on the front stoop said.

"What was this used for?" Alan asked.

He shrugged. "It's been on my wall thirty years. I got it at a yard sale myself."

"I can keep you insured," Bettina said.

"I'd let you keep your job," Alan said, and Bettina smiled.

THEY WERE MARRIED in a morning ceremony two months later. Three accountants attended, and afterward they asked Alan how he got stuck with Bettina after all his beautiful women.

Alan glanced at Bettina, suddenly confused. "Don't talk about my wife that way."

He moved his furniture into the basement of her house. The rooms were full of velvet couches, wooden end tables, and mismatched lamps. The first time Bettina invited Alan over, she'd gone through the rooms telling him which pieces came from her family and which she'd bought at garage sales. He'd found the distinction impossible to guess. When he arrived at the house after the wedding, he discovered that she'd purchased a wheelchair, a recliner with a hydraulic lift, and a hospital bed with collapsible metal sides.

"Your last husband was elderly?" Alan asked.

"You broke it, you buy it." Bettina said.

ALAN FAINTED two more times, he quit his job, and his feet began to swell. When he was feeling well, he dusted the tables and vacuumed between couch cushions. When he was not feeling well, he watched television and read books. His former boss gave him a freelance data entry project that he worked on every morning for an hour to keep busy. Some nights the neighbour couple came over for cards, and Alan was grateful for contact with the outside world.

Bettina left for work at eight o'clock in the morning and was home by five-thirty. She talked about the lab's particle accelerator and the survival rates of heart transplant recipients in the evenings and sang along to the radio as she made dinner while he sat on a dining room chair with a quilt wrapped around him. They turned in early for bed. Alan was nervous about how sex would affect his heart, so Bettina was the centre of his slow attentions. The developing gentleness of his time with her, more than anything his doctor suggested, made Alan certain he wanted a new heart now that he was ill enough to be considered for the transplant list. He talked to his doctor at the university medical centre and was given a beeper.

The beeper rang three times on false alarms during the next two months, but the fourth was a heart coming from Indiana. Alan called Bettina at work, and she drove him to the hospital.

"I hope you get a good one," Bettina said. "What if your donor has bad taste in music?"

"We can retrain it," Alan said. "Like a dog."

BETTINA TOLD HIM LATER that he'd woken up three times after the surgery. He was intubated and she gave him a notebook and pencil when he awoke, wild-eyed and afraid. Each time he wrote on the pad, "How did it go?" It went well, she said. No complications. Alan nodded and collapsed on the pillow. The steroids his doctor prescribed made him hallucinate and he dreamed of oncoming headlights. He woke up when he hit the ground in his dreams.

After he was discharged from the hospital, Alan returned to the couch. He'd gained weight from one of the medicines, so his skin felt puffy and tight, but he was no longer facing the slow approach of death. This time spent at home was convalescence, recovery. His doctor encouraged him to ride a stationary bicycle to improve his endurance, and Bettina purchased one for the living room. Though sore across his rib cage, Alan found that every day he could pedal a bit more. The swelling and weight gain diminished. He went to the hospital for rejection biopsies, and every month the heart seemed resigned to his body.

"When do we start to plan ahead?" Bettina asked, one night after dinner.

"What do you mean?" Alan asked.

"Vacations. Retirement. Children," Bettina said. "Groceries for next week."

"Soon," Alan hesitated. "Soon."

In the first month after his transplant, Alan and Bettina had sex again, but Alan didn't pace himself as he had done when he was ill. He noticed only when he finished that Bettina was looking at him strangely.

"You didn't hardly need me here," she said, getting up from the bed.

Alan watched her walk into the bathroom, and sighed. He did not feel the softness for her that he once felt after they had sex. Since the transplant, he had begun to think of Bettina as a woman who had been kind to him. His disappearing reliance on her, his growing independence, made him feel that he was living with a stranger. He tried to recreate that first conversation with her at the wedding, and now he wondered if their relationship was based on his mistaking disinterest for coyness. She never seemed to be in love with him until he needed her support.

The days at home became interminable for Alan, bicycling, walking around the block, and watching television. He sat in the living room and decided the second-hand furniture made him uncomfortable with its pretension of wisdom and age. Bettina was not surrounding herself in history; she was dull. More than anything, Alan wanted feel to young, as he never had. He wanted the world around him to be full of fresh, untarnished things. On one of his walks around the block, Alan crossed paths with the neighbour woman with whom they'd played cards. She pushed a baby stroller, frowned into the sun, and asked after his health.

"I'm doing better," he said. "How old are your little ones?"

"Eight months," she replied. "I don't like staying at home. I get so bored."

"There are opportunities that an open schedule allows," Alan said.

She smiled at him. Alan wore his undershirt to hide the scar when they had sex in her bed that afternoon, the twins asleep in a playpen.

"Well, that didn't take long," she said, when it was over.

Alan stopped by her house the next week, but she told him she had laundry to do.

"Important laundry," she said. "I need to get to it right now."

THERE WAS ANOTHER housewife, an accounting executive, a nurse at the rehab clinic, and a grocery store clerk. After a sexual encounter with him, women did not want to see Alan again. Even so, his taste for variation had returned. He slept with Bettina out of obligation, though he noticed that she did not dab perfume behind her ears before coming to bed as she once had.

Two months after the transplant, Alan returned to the accounting firm. He did not talk about his new women to the male accountants, because the stories weren't nearly so interesting and he wasn't proud of the encounters as he had been. Alan had a tryst with a secretary in the staff lounge after which she looked at him with that vacant, fearful look he was beginning to recognize as a hallmark of his time with women. After weeks of being healthy for the first time in his life, he began to feel tired and sad. He went to his doctor, thinking that the fatigue might be the first sign of organ rejection, but the doctor confirmed that he was healthy.

BETTINA TOLD ALAN that she wanted to have a garage sale. When she asked him if he would like to help her, he shook his head and did not turn away from the television. Alone, she sat on the couch, decorating posters and writing prices on green stickers she bought at the drugstore and making lists.

"Is there anything that you want to get rid of?" Bettina asked.

Alan shrugged. "Your junk crowds the house."

"You're right," she said. "This place is overcrowded."

On the day of the sale, Alan was gone in the morning with a redhead he'd met at the post office. When he pulled his car up to the house, he saw the hydraulic lift recliner, the wheelchair, his stationary bicycle, and the hospital bed sitting out on the driveway. On the tables were his sweaters and jeans and socks. The furniture that he'd moved into her basement stood on the asphalt. His couch was marked sold. Four people stood around touching his things.

"What is this?" Alan asked, walking up the driveway.

Bettina wore a visor and sat at a card table.

"This thing has run its course," she said.

"Were you going to tell me?" Alan asked.

"You're moving out," Bettina said.

"You're moving me out."

"We had an arrangement, not a marriage."

"I got the transplant because of how happy you made me."

"How happy do I make you now?" Bettina asked.

A woman brought two leather belts to the table. "One dollar each?"

Bettina glanced at Alan. "Sounds fair."

"I don't wear those anymore," he said. The woman gave him two bills. He turned toward Bettina. "I love you. I've grown to love you."

"You're done with me," Bettina said. "I'm just doing the logistical part."

"I hadn't made a decision," Alan said. "I've been out of my head. I think it might be the medicine. Maybe I got the heart of a philanderer. Maybe I need to be retrained. I still need you."

"You don't need me."

"I wish I did," Alan said. "That should count."

"It doesn't. We only love each other in sickness, not in health."

"Can we work on this?" Alan asked.

"You don't do for me as you once did," Bettina said soberly.

Alan looked away. "I don't mean to be unsatisfying."

"You can take a poll. Maybe one of your other ladies will have a different response."

Alan shook his head. "Every woman feels the same. What has changed?"

Bettina frowned. "You could deny the other women out of politeness. Before the transplant, you were insecure and nervous and a little sad and it made you a great lover."

"What am I now?"

"You're as inexperienced as a virgin," Bettina said. "I was the best wife for your affliction. You can have the profits from the garage sale. At least your stuff is out of my house."

ALAN RENTED A ROOM at a motel that night and signed a lease on a one-bedroom apartment the next week. Bettina filed for divorce, and the marriage was over in a matter of months. He missed her presence in his life at first, but he quickly fell into new routines and began to plan a backpack trip to Australia and applied for a bachelor's degree in business. At night he dreamed of oncoming headlights and beautiful women. He tried to remember how he had pleased the women of his past, what he had slowed down that other men rushed, but he could not. He had lost the discipline of illness, the way it allowed him to focus on the smallest of desires. He regretted the loss of this concentration, of course, but with the future before him, he hadn't time to worry over any pleasure but his own.

Lorie Kolak was awarded first prize in the 2007 Goldenberg Fiction Contest, sponsored by Bellevue Literary Review. She works at DePaul University library and lives in Chicago.

My Little Heart Attack

Tom Lombardo

went by so fast
it didn't stop my singing
or my dancing with my children—
twirling Sam and Lucy's tiny hands
around my fingers, their long hair flying
until ventricular tachycardia
at two too many beats per measure
sat me down to rest my chest.
I took my tricky heart to Dr. Takahachi's office.
He said, "Let me palpate
your thorax. Breathe. Yes. Copasetic."

Someone else called nine one one

when myocardial infarction
hiding in my warty arteries
started stallions galloping across my sternum
until EMS responded, pounded
K-Y Jelly into my ribs,
convulsed me repeatedly
with portable defibrillator paddles
while I danced and twirled
their little hands, "Again! Again!"
they called like Sam and Lucy
denying it's time for bed.

Tom Lombardo's poems have appeared in many literary journals. He holds his MFA in creative writing, has been a journalist for twenty years, and teaches creative writing.

The Eighth Day

Michael Constantine McConnell

I'd been in the hospital for several days, enduring test after test in the afternoons. Doctors had taped wires to my wrists, wires that sent lightning up my arm; they'd put me inside of a tube-shaped machine that made horrible clanging-metal loud sounds around my head. They'd poked and pricked needle after needle into my arms and fingers. They'd given me cup after cup of acrid-tasting medicine to drink because I didn't know how to swallow pills and would gag when I tried. The doctors would start every day in the late morning, and they would test me until about four in the afternoon, long after I'd become exhausted.

I lay on the bed one evening, watching the television in one of the ceiling-corners of my hospital room. My mother had left to get something for dinner, promising me that she'd return as soon as she was done eating. I watched TV while falling in and out of sleep. A doctor walked into my room.

"Hello, Michael," he said, holding a clipboard in one hand and a white towel, glinting with shiny metal instruments, in the other hand. "How are you feeling?"

"Okay," I slowly mumbled, my consciousness continuing to totter slightly between sleep and waking. I looked at the shiny little metallic teeth bundled up in the towel. The doctor put his clipboard on the table next to my bed.

"I need you to roll over," he said, resting the towel on the bed next to me, the little metal instruments tapping against each other like barely audible wind chimes. I shifted my weight and tried to roll over, but I couldn't without the doctor's help. He placed one hand on my waist and the other on my shoulder, pushing me over on my side.

"What are you going to do?" I asked. Every day, the doctors would help motivate me through the painful and exhausting tests by telling me that there were only a few left, that there were only three tests, two tests, one test left, and after the last test, they'd tell me that I was finished for the day, that I wouldn't have to do anymore until tomorrow.

"Micheal," he said. "You are going to have to stay very still."

"Okay," I said, turning my head so that I could watch the television while the doctor did whatever he was about to do. He untied and pulled my gown open, and I felt something cold and wet against the skin on my lower back. I flinched.

"Michael," the doctor sternly said, "I have to give you a spinal tap. If you move while I'm doing this, if you so much as cough, you may never walk again. Now, stay still and try to relax."

I held my breath. My weak body went completely limp. Although I stared straight ahead, I couldn't see anything. In the very depths of my mind stood a colossal mountain with a fat little boy sitting calmly on its peak and looking out over serene dreamscape, and inside of that fat little boy's mind stood another colossal mountain with another fat little boy sitting on its peak and looking out over an even more serene dreamscape, and so on, and in the very centre of it all existed coldness and darkness, and I trembled in this place while listening to the ugly sound and ignoring the horrifying feeling of a needle wiggling around the bones of my lower back.

"Good job," the doctor said, retying the strings on the back of my gown. "You can turn back over now." He gently pulled my waist and shoulder, rolling me onto my back. I heard his footsteps grow faint as he walked out of the room, and suddenly the ceiling came into focus. I turned my head, I wiggled my fingers, but I didn't breathe until one of the machines next to my bed sounded a loud shrill, beeping alarm—a common sound in the Children's Hospital intensive care ward—and a nurse ran into the room.

"Michael," she said, pressing a button on the machine and turning off the alarm. "Don't hold your breath like that; this isn't a game." I didn't answer. With my breathing came sobbing.

"Honey," she said, "what's wrong? Why are you crying?" I tried to speak, to say that I wanted to go home, that I didn't want to be in a wheelchair for the rest of my life, but the words turned into sand in my mouth.

After the first week, the doctors told my mother that I'd contracted Guillain-Barré syndrome, a virus that attacks the nervous system. For the past week, I'd twitch at the feeling of fire on my skin, fire that wasn't there. I'd wince at the feeling of absent needles piercing my bones and muscles. The entire lower half of my body, from my the top of my thighs to the tips of my feet, felt like somebody or something had grabbed all ten of my toes, crushed them into each other, and twisted them like the key on a wind-up toy until my legs formed a tight spiral.

I could move my arms but had limited control. My muscles were weak, and I'd lost much balance and hand-to-eye coordination. For dinner one night, the nurse had served me a sloppy joe, one of my favourite meals. I picked up the sandwich with both weak hands and lifted it to my open mouth, missing completely and smearing tomato sauce and loose meat all over my cheeks and nose. My mother cleaned my face and fed the rest of the meal to me by hand. After that, she hand-fed every meal to me, bite by bite, spoon to mouth.

I tried time and time again to tell my mother and the doctors and nurses that the cherry pie from Andy's had made me sick, but the doctors reassured me that a person couldn't contract Guillain-Barré through food or drinks, nor could one person catch if from someone else. They explained that the rare disease affects one in every hundred thousand people and that there was nothing anyone could have done to foresee it or prevent me from catching it. They said I would most likely recover fully from the disease, but that my condition would worsen before it improved, and it could take as little as a few months or as many as five or ten years to get better.

Every day, different members of my family would come to see me during evening visiting hours. On some days, my mother would bring Nunie to visit me. On some days, my Aunt Mary Anne would visit. On some days, my Uncle Tommy would visit with his friend Brad, and they'd kneel by my bed, holding my hands and praying aloud to God for my recovery. Sometimes Matt, the downstairs neighbour, would visit, reading comic books to me and showing me the colourful pictures.

Although I appreciated all of my visitors and every toy and stuffed animal they'd bring me, I became especially excited when Aunt Caroline brought her husband Rick with her. Rick was my hero, and I wanted to grow up and be just like him. I wanted to be bigger than life, with long hair, a thick beard, and arms covered with tattoos of flaming skulls. One night he gave me a metal sheriff's badge, telling me that it was real, that an actual sheriff had worn it.

My mother visited me daily. After working the morning shift at her waitressing job at a Coney Island restaurant, she'd drive straight to the hospital, greeting me with a strong smile and reeking of chili dogs and mustard. She'd stay by my side for the rest of the day, holding my hand between tests and feeding my meals to me. The nurses let her stay with me after visiting hours, and she'd play with me. I always wanted to play "Sheriff," so she'd pin the badge to my gown and wheel me through the halls. Whenever we found an empty hallway, I'd say, "Let's get the bad guys, Mommy," and she would push me while she ran, gaining speed then slowing to a stop so that we wouldn't crash into a wall. I would laugh, shooting imaginary criminals with my index fingers, and say, "Do it again, Mommy, do it again—faster, faster."

I can't imagine my mother's side of this story, the agony that she must have felt seeing me in that condition. She was a single mother, and I was all that she had. Despite the hardship of watching her little boy's health deteriorating, she remained strong in my presence and always spoke hopefully about my recovery, even when I was at my sickest and weakest, when the doctors told her that they'd have to give me a tracheotomy and pump oxygen into my lungs so that I wouldn't stop breathing in the middle of the night. After the evenings of playing "Sheriff" with me, she'd put me to bed and sit in a chair next to me for hours. Because of the awkward, painful, and uncomfortable sensations I'd feel in my legs and feet, I couldn't sleep very well, but I'd lie completely still in bed, pretending to sleep while she sobbed herself to sleep. I'd usually fall asleep after a nurse came in and covered my mother with a blanket.

Fortunately, I never had to have the tracheotomy. Like the doctors had said, my condition worsened, but after about ten days in the hospital, I made a private choice. I told myself that I was tired of being in a wheelchair, unable to walk. I wanted to run and jump and walk like a normal child, and I vowed that I wouldn't let Guillain-Barré syndrome win the battle. I remember the day, the moment, when I willed the wretched disease to leave me alone forever. When I made the choice, I'd already completed the diagnostic phase of my visit, so I didn't have to take any more tests, which gave me more time to spend in the playroom. I'd gotten better at manoeuvring my wheelchair, so I snuck away from the playroom when the nurse on duty wasn't looking, and I quickly wheeled myself to the visitors lobby, which stayed empty until the evening visiting hours. I sat alone in the empty room, pushing my hands against the armrests to raise my butt off the wheelchair, then I relaxed and my butt dropped back down. I repeated the process until my arms hurt, then I wheeled myself back to the playroom unnoticed.

I snuck away and practised standing up every day, and each time I progressed further. On the second day, I raised my butt out of the wheelchair, locked my elbows, and pushed against the ground with my weak legs, rocking my torso back and forth like a swing. On the third day, I lifted my butt out of the chair and, holding tightly to the armrests, took small steps forward and backward and to the side. On the fourth day, I pushed myself into a standing position, then fell back into the chair. On the fifth day, I stood for two seconds without holding onto the chair. On the sixth day, I took one step forward before falling back into the chair. On the seventh day, I took two steps.

The eighth day was Valentine's Day, February 14, 1979. My grade 1 teacher from Robinson Elementary visited me, and she gave me a bag of chocolate hearts and dozens of letters that my classmates had written, telling me to get better soon so that I could come back to school and play. After she left, I wheeled myself to the nurse station in the centre of the fourth floor, where all hallways converged. The nurses threw us a party, and they'd covered the walls with paper hearts and hung red streamers across the ceiling. My mother had told me the day before that she'd probably be late for the party because of work but that she would be there, and she never let me down on such promises. I sat patiently, biding my time and waiting to show her a secret that belonged only to me.

After I'd waited for about forty-five minutes, eating chocolate hearts and reading my classmates' letters, I saw my mother walk into the nurse station area, holding a bouquet of flowers and a box of chocolates. I pushed myself up with my arms and stood shakily in front of the wheelchair that had substituted as my legs for over two weeks. A hush fell over the floor and drop-jawed nurses stepped out of the path of my mother, who had dropped the bouquet of flowers and a box of chocolates on the floor at her feet. I swung my body and lifted one of my legs, catching my weight and balance when my foot retouched the ground. I took another step. I wasn't holding on to the wheelchair anymore, and the world advanced in slow motion. I took another step. I looked up. My mother held her hands out to me, motioning for me to walk the rest of the way, assuring me that everything was going to be all right. Tears poured in steady streams out of her eyes. I lunged out a few more jerky steps and collapsed into her arms.

"Happy Valentine's Day, Mommy."

She dropped to her knees, holding me, crying, and hugging me tightly. I could feel her tears on my hospital gown. I could feel tears streaming down my cheeks. I looked up at the tear-filled faces of the nurses who had surrounding us and placed their hands on our shoulders. One of the nurses moved to the side and grabbed my arm, shaking it. I looked up at her, and she smiled at me and pointed to a doctor standing about ten feet away.

"Michael," the nurse said, wiping her eyes with her shirt collar, "can you show him what you just showed us?" My mother lifted her head off my neck and kissed every part of my face, holding my cheeks in her hands. She looked at the nurse, then at the doctor. She gave me another tight hug and stood up, holding onto my arms so that I wouldn't fall.

"Go ahead, Michael," she said with a happier smile on her face than I've ever seen. "Walk to him." She held lightly onto my wrists, helping me keep my balance, then let go after I started walking. I lifted my feet and stepped one at a time, wobbling on my legs and waving my arms, but I didn't fall. I walked into my doctor's outstretched arms, and he picked me up, carried me across the room, and put me back into my wheelchair.

"Well, Ms. Piggins," the doctor said to my mother. "You've got quite the little fighter on your hands, don't you?"

"Yes, I do," said my mother, sniffling and wiping her nose with her shirtsleeve.

"I've seen some amazing recoveries," he said. "But I've never seen anything like that. Not with Guillain-Barré."

I spent the rest of the afternoon laughing, playing with the other children, and eating chocolate. Although the nurses told my mother not to let me eat too much, she let me eat chocolate until my lips and tongue turned brown. That night, we played "Sheriff," our favourite game, and as my mother ran down the hallway pushing me in my wheelchair, I knew that soon I'd be running next to her.

Michael McConnell, of Denton, TX, is a writer of poems, prose, and palindromes, Experimental Word Forms editor for Farrago's Wainscot *(www.farragoswainscot.com), and a student of the upright bass, piano, autoharp, and twenty-button Anglo concertina.*

Life Study

Helen McLean

I've been looking with renewed interest at a work that's been hanging on my living room wall for the past twenty-odd years. It's a drawing by the late Erik Loder, a painter and consummately talented draughtsman whom I knew during the dozen years I lived in the country near Peterborough, Ontario. The work is executed in black crayon on white paper, with a few strokes of red and some smudges of violet to emphasize roundness of contour and areas of shadow. The model is a young girl who stands turned away from the viewer, so the right side of her face and one breast and the gentle curve of her belly are in profile. In the three-quarter view of her back, both shoulders and the elbow of the far arm and all of the near arm can be seen. Her muscles are supple-looking and unexaggerated, the hips slim, buttocks rounded. A few lines on the lower part of the drawing represent folds of drapery, as though the model had allowed a wrapper or gown to slide down to below her hips where she now holds it against either thigh with her hands.

But there's more. Within the figure's outline Loder has drawn and shaded in parts of the girl's skeleton—the neck bones, the vertebrae of the spine, the bones of the nearer upper arm and forearm and the neatly articulated projection of the elbow; a shoulder blade, a slab of ribs, the pelvis where it joins the lower end of the backbone—all without any sense of the macabre or feeling that the work was intended sardonically as a memento mori. When I bought the drawing from Erik all those years ago, I asked him if, during the course of his studies in New York, he'd been required to work from the skeleton and from those flayed figures that expose the musculature of the human body. He replied, "Of course," sounding surprised by the question, as though such exercises would have been part of any art-school curriculum. He went on to say that he included bones in many of his life-studies because he particularly liked drawing them, and after all it was the bones that gave the body its form, the way foundations and beams are what give its final shape to a house.

Bones have been very much on my mind lately. If I were to use Erik's fanciful simile and liken my own bones to the foundations and beams of the fleshly house in which my spirit dwells, I would say that the building had begun to go askew, that the beams and foundations were showing signs of deterioration that was causing a sagging and a listing and a painful grating of the hinges.

A specialist I consulted told me the problem was one that had to be taken seriously: the supporting timbers were no longer sound or true and the whole edifice was being thrown out of kilter. No makeshift propping up would do, either. The place was old, in case I hadn't noticed; in real-estate lingo it would be called a heritage property. Things were not going to right themselves on their own, either. What was happening now could only get worse, and would certainly do so if the situation were ignored. Fortunately there were modern methods for restoring old frameworks like mine. A rotten beam and joist could be cut away and discarded and a metal jack and other parts installed in their place to set the structure in line again. In his skilful hands and with the use of the best modern materials the renovations would last—quick glance to check my date of birth—my lifetime.

At the clinic they took X-rays, and parts of me I'd never seen before—or what I was told were parts of me (I wasn't convinced they hadn't mixed my pictures up with someone else's)—were put up on the computer screen. Severe osteoarthritis of the right hip, the only cure: total hip replacement. *Total hip replacement?* Whoa there! Just a darn minute! Yes, of course I'd been having discomfort walking, that was why I was here. All right, *severe* discomfort. Yes, I suppose you could call it pain. Getting into the car was a bit of a hassle, but I'd gotten used to lifting the leg with both hands and hauling it in after me so that wasn't a real problem, but I would admit that climbing the stairs was becoming a pain in the neck, I mean the hip. The man in charge tapped on the screen with a pencil.

Look. See. Right there. The cartilage has all worn away, the lubricating juices have dried up, the hip socket and the ball on the head of the femur are all frayed and scruffy. The joint's worn out. What you've got there is bone grating on bone.

When I got home I did some Internet research about the surgery I'd just agreed to undergo. I turned up what looked to be a reliable article on the subject, but found I couldn't read it all at once without breaking out in a sweat and having my hair stand on end, so I downloaded it and decided to absorb it in gradual doses over a period of time.

The steps for replacing the hip begin with making an incision about eight inches long over the hip joint. After the incision is made, the ligaments and muscles are separated to allow the surgeon access to the bones of the hip joint. Once the hip joint is entered, the femoral head is dislocated from the acetabulum. Then the femoral head is removed by cutting through the femoral neck with a power saw.[1]

The brochure showed the parts in question in the form of simple diagrams. I imagined the details for myself—the clamps and vises, the pipewrenches and hacksaw blades, the spattering blood and the bone chips flying through the air.

I don't know with any degree of accuracy how the bones of the human body articulate with one another, where the muscles attach, how an arm or a leg works. My artistic education, unlike Erik Loder's, was somewhat hit and miss. Much as I love drawing and painting the human figure, my knowledge of its mechanics is rudimentary, and any skeleton I might draw would look like a decoration for a kids' Halloween party. A lot of paper still gets wasted when I draw, and much trial and error lies buried under layers of paint on my canvases. During my early student days I learned a few schemas for making parts of the body look plausible, like sectioning off a basic egg shape for a head and getting the features in more or less the right places by setting the eyes halfway between crown

---

1. Medical Multimedia Group, "A Patient's Guide to Artificial Replacement of the Hip," eorthopod, http://www.eorthopod.com/public/patient_education/6493/artificial_joint_replacement_of_the_hip.html (accessed July 31, 2007).

and chin. I recall being taught in high-school art classes how to measure a standing figure into an appropriate seven or eight "heads," to put a man's navel at his waist and a woman's a little lower on the abdomen, to have the legs account for half the average person's height. The classrooms were full of live human beings of which any one might easily have served as a model for the rest, but at that early stage of our artistic education few if any of us were ready for drawing from life. We hadn't learned the language yet, did not know how to reconfigure in our heads what our eyes were seeing and translate it into intelligible marks on the paper. Arriving at that level takes a great deal of study and practice.

If you give a three-year-old paper and crayons and ask him to make a picture of a tree, he doesn't run to the window to look at the maple on the front lawn, he draws what he already knows about trees and produces a green lollipop on a brown stick. It would be nice to think that all budding artists have to do is grab pencil and paper and learn everything they need to know by looking at what's in front of their eyes, but before a painter can even begin to develop an individual style by which his work may later be identified, he has to bring the overwhelmingly complex natural world under control by devising and storing up a repository of abstract templates, like the child's lollipop tree. In his book *Art and Illusion* art historian and theorist Ernst Gombrich quotes Nietzsche, who said that since nature can't be subdued by the artist, he chooses from it what he likes, and paints that. And what does he like? Why, what he knows how to paint—which will be the things that have caught his attention and he has developed the skill to represent—like Erik Loder with his figures and bones.

Special rasps are used to shape and hollow out the femur to the exact shape of the metal stem of the femoral component. Once the size and shape of the canal exactly fit the femoral component, the stem is inserted into the femur . . . the stem is held in place by the tightness of the fit into the bone (similar to the friction that holds a nail driven into a hole drilled into wooden board—with a slightly smaller diameter than the nail).[2]

Gombrich calls it the modern dilemma that the developing of a schematic vocabulary has been thrown out of art-school curricula, leaving

---

2. Ibid.

the artist high and dry. High and dry, and, one might add, as blissfully free as a toddler on the beach flinging sand in every direction. The old sine qua non of the artist as being someone who knows how to draw has been tossed aside. "Creativity" (a word that makes me flinch) is thought to lie within every breast, and for those who can't discover their own vein of the precious lode there is no shortage of workshops offering to give the process a kick start. What Umberto Eco calls an orgy of tolerance is in mode, a bland all-inclusiveness that lacks even the wryness of Dada or the irony of camp.

Those in favour of the kind of painting that makes no reference to the visible world argue that the work itself is an object in the visible world and as such is not required to represent or even refer to anything else. Fair enough, but curators and gallery-owners and artists themselves seem unwilling to leave it at that. Lest the work and the circumstances of its conception be misinterpreted, they print up and post alongside it lengthy tracts about the artist's philosophy, his intentions, and his psychic state at the time of painting, often in language so turgid as to make one wonder if it's actually about the painting in question. One such commentary doesn't necessarily jibe with the next. Barnett Newman's jumbo tri-colour canvas *Voice of Fire* in Canada's National Gallery was described in the accompanying literature as "an objectification of thought that floods our consciousness with a sublime sense of awe and tranquility," while elsewhere the same painting was said to represent "the anguish of man's abandonment." Take your pick.

When there are no clues as to what the artist wanted the viewer to take from a work, everyone who looks at it will dredge up something from his own experience and project it onto the painting, deciphering its forms as mattress ticking or flying tiddlywinks or a chicken's viscera. If that kind of subjective reading was the artist's intention, fine, but if he really wants to get his own point of view across it's no fair breaking into print to do it. There's a whole world out there for him to weld his ideas to, whether it be forms from nature or esoteric icons or commonplace objects, like the pots and bottles Giorgio Morandi managed to infuse with so much mystery and metaphysical meaning. Cézanne chose apples and a blue-and-white ginger pot and the faceted slopes of Mont Ste. Victoire as the framework for his formal discoveries, probably for no other reason than that he enjoyed painting them. I doubt whether artistic talent, where it actually exists, is so fragile a flower that it shrivels under exposure to diligent instruction. The compulsion to make art is not easy to repress or divert, and it would be better, I think, to have mastered a repertoire of schemas and procedures against which to rebel, or to revise to suit one's needs, or in the end discard altogether, than to be cast rudderless into a sea of benign permissiveness.

In the uncemented variety of artificial hip replacement, the metal shell is simply held in place by the tightness of the fit or with screws to hold the metal shell in place.[3]

Among my late mother's childhood keepsakes (she was born in rural Ontario in 1901) I found a doll, a baby's form reduced to the simplest of schemas—seven round wooden balls of graduated sizes strung together on a cord, with a tiny ball on either side of the largest one for ears. The toy is of a size to fit small hands, and it bends and nods just enough to give it a semblance of life and motion. It has no arms or legs as such—this baby is obviously swaddled, so the bottom end of it comes more or less to a point, like Popeye's "adoptid infink" Swee'Pea—and the face has no features unless you count those ears, but even a tiny child would know what it represents. We project what we want to see, which is most often an image of our own kind, and we manage to find it on the moon or on the knotty trunk of a tree, a decayed masonry wall, or in a blob on a toasted cheese sandwich. Perhaps all earthly creatures seek others of their own species to reassure themselves that they're not alone in the universe—like my dog who becomes exhilarated at the sight of another dog a hundred yards away across a grassy field. I am no exception. When a human figure appears in a work of art, even a tiny one in a very large painting, to it my eye flies first. I'm with Auden who wrote,

> To me art's subject is the human clay
> And landscape but a background to a torso.
> All Cézanne's apples I would give away
> For one small Goya or a Daumier.[4]

---

3. Ibid.
4. Auden, W. H. *Letter to Lord Byron*, edited by Edward Mendelson (London: Faber & Faber), 100.

Lucian Freud admits to harbouring a little of the Pygmalion fantasy, a barely conscious hope that some day one of his painted figures might actually come to life. He has said that when it becomes obvious that a work close to completion is turning out to be just another picture after all, he feels let down. If ever a painted figure were to draw breath and step down off the canvas it would be one of Freud's, but probably most figurative artists feel a little God-like when a new work is getting under way, when the image is still immanent and the painting can become almost anything wished for. If actual life can't be imparted to a painted figure, there can be another kind of life in the work as a whole, an aesthetic quality that infuses it with electric energy. When Erik Loder wasn't drawing his eloquent half-transparent nudes he turned his attention to what was growing in his garden and drew huge cabbages that were ready to burst, or sprawling clumps of rhubarb shooting their seed-stalks skyward with such force one could almost hear them screech.

You now have a new weight-bearing surface to replace your diseased hip. The therapist will carefully instruct you on how to avoid activities and positions which increase the risk of hip dislocation.[5]

The structure now requires only the support of a single flying buttress, and even that becomes less and less necessary as weeks pass. Until recently I never gave a thought to canes or the people who carried them. My father sported one in his younger days for purely ornamental purposes—during the thirties a slender brass-ferruled cane was a dandyish Burlington Bertie accessory to be swung forward and allowed to hit the ground only at every other step—a balletic manoeuvre that distinguished the debonair from the disabled. My father-in-law on the other hand, whom I knew only in his later years, was a serious walker, and would sally forth on a brisk four- or five-mile hike of a Sunday afternoon having made a selection (usually a gnarled blackthorn) from an assortment of sturdy walking sticks kept in a polished brass stand in the vestibule. Now that the snow has melted and we of unsteady step are able to venture out of doors, I'm surprised to note that I pass half a dozen other cane-users during a stroll of only a few blocks, many of us women and all

---

5. Medical Multimedia Group.

of us vintage to a greater or lesser degree. There's a sort of camaraderie among cane-users—we nod to each other or raise our walking sticks in greeting as we pass, perhaps saluting one another's continuing mobility.

Hopefully, you can expect 12–15 years of service from your artificial hip.[6]

That ought to do it.

When I was a young child at the Loretto day-school in Toronto, Mother Maureen used to lead our Grade 4 class in prayer each morning, asking God for the quick release from purgatory of the soul that was closest to heaven. We were convinced of the strength and effectiveness of our supplications, certain that if we all prayed like sixty the transfer would occur immediately, with a sound like a popping cork. After a long cold Toronto winter, my whole being yearns for spring, but I no longer pray for specific results, and in any case I know that yanking the new season up from below the American border into this temperate just-right latitude would be well beyond my spiritual powers. Yearn as I might, I don't expect to get up one morning and find that all the trees in the park and on the hillside are suddenly green with fresh new leaves just because I want them to be. I do however take careful notice of their miniscule day-by-day changes.

Gombrich says perceiving is not the same as seeing, that perceiving is an active process that should more properly be called noticing. We look, he says, when our attention is aroused, and only then do we notice that things aren't the way they were before, or as we expected them to be. Over a period of several days of intense observation from my eighth-floor balcony I thought I could detect an incremental thickening of the skeletal upper branches of the trees in the park. One morning there even seemed to be a decidedly purplish-pink colour in the crown of the great copper beech, so I went down on the elevator and out the front door and around the corner to the park and stood leaning against that massive trunk, staring upward. Sure enough, at the very tips of the highest branches little pointed red leaves were beginning to appear. I looked

---

6. Ibid.

around and saw that tiny bright green blossoms were beginning to burst forth on the lower grey branches of the neighbouring maple tree.

As though to confirm my observations, a rosy-headed house finch swooped down and landed on the back of one of the wooden park benches, trilled a few notes, and took off again.

Helen McLean has followed a dual career as an artist and writer. She is the author of two novels, two memoirs, and a collection of essays. Her novel Significant Things *was shortlisted for the 2004 Commonwealth Writer's Prize, Canada/Caribbean division. Her paintings are in many private and public collections, including the Margaret Laurence Home in Neepawa, Manitoba, and the Bank of Canada, Ottawa. Recent articles, reviews, and essays have appeared in* The Globe and Mail, Brick, *the* National Post, Books in Canada, Literary Review of Canada, Quill & Quire, Room of One's Own, Ars Medica, *and* Accenti Magazine. *Her books include* Sketching From Memory: A Portrait of My Mother *(Oberon, 1994),* Of All the Summers *(Women's Press, 1999),* Details from a Larger Canvas *(Dundurn Press, 2001),* Significant Things: A Novel *(Dundurn Press, 2003), and* Just Looking and Other Essays *(Seraphim Editions, 2008).*

Second Sight

Helen McLean

Plato was probably right when he said that the root of artistic creation was an inspired madness. Artists can be obsessives, driven human beings who can't entertain the thought of quitting even when they're overtaken by old age and infirmity. During his last years Renoir painted with his brushes strapped to hands gnarled with arthritis; aged and half-blind Monet combined pigments from memory while he painted one of the major masterpieces of his life. Bonnard lay on his deathbed directing his niece who was looking after him where to dab a few more brush-loads of colour on what turned out to be his final painting. But it's not only geniuses who are obsessed. As a non-genius painter, even I can't imagine still being on this earth and not wanting to draw and paint. Maybe the way to bring on real craziness is to prevent an artist from working.

Art was never Plato's favourite thing anyway. In his view anything from the natural world, a pot of geraniums, say, is sandwiched between an immaterial Ideal Form of geraniums of which the plant itself is already an imitation, and the final imitation that is the artist's image. To him art was at worst a dangerous delusion and at best an entertainment. Here Plato and I part company. I think an artist's goal and what fuels his or her desire is neither to translate into material form some abstract concept of Beauty nor to make a lifelike copy of that wretched pot of geraniums, but something else entirely. I have never begun a painting or even a drawing without first having had not only a fleeting vision in my mind's eye of how the finished work will (or should) look but what kind of emotion it will arouse in me when I see it. That moment of intuition is not only what sets me going but is the standard by which I will judge the piece at the end. While there is the rare euphoria-inducing occasion when it seems almost impossible to make a wrong brush stroke, most of the time I only come close to where I want to go and frequently fail altogether. The thing may be well enough executed but it will have a kind of slackness, a lack of energy and compression, so that the feeling is weakly expressed or missing altogether. The strange part is that, far from discouraging me, my failures egg me on to start anew and this time get it right, so around I go again.

Where the fleeting vision comes from that stamps itself so firmly on my mind's eye is a mystery, but what is certain is that it calls the shots, and if the phenomenon is as universal as I believe it to be it shows no more mercy toward the genius than to the artist of small talent. Cézanne wrestled through more than a hundred sittings for which the dealer Ambroise Vollard patiently posed before the artist finally abandoned the project, remarking, as he tossed down his brushes and shoved the canvas into a corner, that he was not entirely displeased with the shirt-front. No one but Cézanne himself could know what he found unsatisfactory about that never-finished painting.

Not that eyesight of the ordinary kind doesn't affect an artist's work. I have read that the figures in El Greco's monumental works may have been so strangely elongated because he had astigmatism and that Monet probably used so much blue in his later paintings because that was one of the few colours he could still see. From my own recent experience I've begun to wonder whether Claude Lorraine suffered from cataracts, if he painted all his romantic Italian landscapes bathed in a golden-umber light because that was the way he saw them.

For my part I prefer blue Italian skies to look blue, or rather that colour into which our eyes translate empty space, but over a period of two or three years I became aware that an ochre cloud was dulling the colour of my own Canadian skies, darkening the page I was reading, smudging my drawings, and fogging the words on my computer screen. The cataracts were at first a nuisance, and then a trial, and finally an intolerable despoiler of everything my eyes fell upon. The ophthalmologist I consulted showed me a little bottle of formaldehyde containing the cataracted lens from a human eye. It looked like a bead of tapioca dipped in coffee or dabbed with yellow-brown paint. No wonder my view of the world was jaundiced. I <u>decided to go ahead</u> and have the surgery he recommended, even though the thought of letting someone go at my eyes with a knife was, to say the least, daunting.

I arrived at the hospital early in the morning during the tail end of Toronto's outbreak of severe acute respiratory syndrome. Did I have fever, chills, a cough, or difficulty breathing? No. Was anyone in my family ill? No. Had I visited another health-care facility during the past two weeks? No. I was handed a mask and told to clean my hands with antiseptic gel.

Upstairs in the Day Surgery Department I was shown to a cubicle, told to take everything off and put on two cotton hospital gowns, one forward and one backward, plus plastic shower cap, paper shoes, and another mask. A plastic ID bracelet was fastened to my wrist. In a waiting area I was assigned a comfortable Archie Bunker chair with extending footrest and a kindly person wrapped a warmed flannelette sheet around me. Two other capped and masked patients tucked up in their own chairs had been watching me settle in; we smiled at one another by crinkling our eyes.

That I was nervous as a cat showed in my elevated blood pressure when they took it. Today's surgery would be on my right eye, the one most seriously afflicted, and several kinds of drops were now put into it, of which some stung mightily. A needle with a syringe tube attached was inserted into a vein in the back of my hand, capped off and taped down. In due time an orderly came to lead me and the two other patients, all of us trailing our blankies, down a corridor, onto an elevator, off again on a higher floor and through a pair of doors marked DO NOT ENTER, at which point he was relieved of his charges and we were shown to another waiting area.

A nurse carrying a clipboard sat down beside each of us in turn, checking things off. Was this my signature giving consent to the operation? I was without my glasses, so I couldn't actually read anything because of the rotten vision in one eye and the other being completely out of it from the drops, but I said yes. Was I allergic to anything, did I have diabetes, could I climb a flight of stairs, could I—not would I, but could I—tell her my date of birth? Yes I could: six-six-twenty-seven I said smartly. She checked that off, stood up, took my arm, and led me through another set of doors into a brilliantly lit room where a group of masked and gowned people were standing around a white-sheeted table. Among them I recognized my eye doctor, who greeted me and helped me onto the table.

I lay there with nothing to do while they fussed around with equipment. They stuck some leads on me here and there and I noticed with bemused interest that a rhythmic beeping from somewhere behind my head was cleverly coinciding with the beating of my heart. A spurt of cold liquid went shooting up my forearm through the needle in the back of my hand and seconds later I felt a spreading warmth, like the first good swallow of a straight up extra-dry martini. Now they were rolling the lid of my right eye up on something, a handy matchstick perhaps, so I couldn't close it any more—but no matter, someone began sluicing the eye comfortably with tepid water.

I sighed deeply, without moving of course, just to let them know I was still in there. Suddenly a dark tunnel appeared in my field of vision and at the end of it, a dazzling white light. If I was being launched on that final journey through space and time to where Glory awaits, I thought, I'd better pay close attention in case I wanted to describe it later to some old friend in the next world. There was a little intermittent whirring noise, like a dentist's drill with the sound turned away down. Kaleidoscopic colours and lights appeared, sparkled and fragmented and reassembled. More whirring. More lights, more colours, some red, some blue, some a blurry mixture. No pain, no pressure, just a sense that things were going on close to where I lived.

I had a pretty good idea of what was happening because I'd read up on it ahead of time. The doctor had made a tiny incision in my eye where the coloured part meets the white, through which he inserted an ultrasound-tipped probe to break apart the cataract and then vacuum out the pieces, leaving behind the little cup called a posterior capsule in which the natural lens used to sit. In the olden days surgery had to wait until the cataract had matured, or ripened, as they called it, which really meant hardened to the point that it could be plucked out like a dried pea. In the days before the invention of modern suturing materials the eye had to heal on its own while the patient lay abed, head sandbagged down to keep from shifting around and disrupting the healing. Sutures were used later, but even then, with no lens in the eye to focus light onto the retina, the patient would have to wear bottle-bottom glasses forever. Nowadays implanted lenses are made-to-measure for the customer from space-age plastics and the incision is shaped in such a way that the fluid pressure inside the eye miraculously seals it shut without the need for any sutures at all.

When it was over, a nurse helped me to sit up on the edge of the table and I perched there for a moment, collecting myself. She stood in front of me, steadying me with a gentle hand on my shoulder, and to my freshly hatched eye, even with its enormously dilated pupil and overflow of fogging tears, her gown was the most astonishing blue I had ever seen, a blue so remarkable that I closed the new eye and looked at this phenomenon with my other, unoperated-upon eye. There was the blue I'd become accustomed to over the years, a dulled down greenish-brownish melancholy blue with all the power drained out of it, the blues of the Sistine Chapel ceiling before the layers of varnish and dirt were cleaned away.

Back home, still drowsy, I flopped down on the sofa between the windows in the dining room. My glance fell on a blue pitcher on the serving table across the room, a kitchen item really, but its colour and shape are appealing so I keep it in view and use it occasionally as a vase for flowers. I stared. What was it with blue? Like that nurse's gown, the pitcher was so blue I could have wept for its blueness, could have dived into that blue and submerged myself in it, been absorbed by it. It was a cerulean sort of hue but with a little more purple to it, maybe a touch of cobalt or ultramarine but not enough to make it dark or turn it into the kind of blue that backs away and lets other colours take precedence. This blue was right here, present, on the surface of the air, like the blues in one of Bonnard's paintings of the descending terraces at Le Cannet, with their red roofs and palms and pines and finally the distant azure sea, and above it all a great arc of the infinite Mediterranean sky. His last canvas, painted at the age of eighty, was of an almond tree in bloom against just such a sky, just such a blue.

Monet was seventy-two when he was diagnosed with cataracts in both eyes. He was offered surgery, beginning with the eye most badly afflicted, but was afraid to undergo it in case he lost his sight in the eye entirely. I could sympathize. Even as I walked into the operating room

I wondered if some unexpected anomaly would crop up and I'd end up worse off than I was before. I could still see, after all, even if what I saw was blurred and tarnished. When Monet faced his decision in 1912, there were no antibiotics to prevent or combat infection, no steroid drops to reduce swelling, no cunning stitchless self-closing incisions, no lasers, no ultrasound probes. He turned it down.

Eleven years later his vision had degenerated to the point that it was virtually non-existent in the right eye and there was only 10 per cent remaining in the left. With so little sight in that right eye he figured he had nothing to lose. He entered the clinic in Neuilly and underwent surgery, after which the eye was kept bandaged for ten days and another twenty days passed before he was fitted with corrective glasses. As it turned out the surgery helped with his close vision but the distance vision remained far from good, and colours were elusive. Later, when a celebrated ophthalmologist visited him at Giverny and asked how his eyes were coming along, Monet said, *"Je vois bleu, mais je ne vois plus le rouge, je ne vois plus le jaune."*

Now, in order to paint with colours he could no longer see, he chose them by their names on the tubes, mixing the pigments in the proportions he knew would produce the oranges and greens and violets, the rosy hues and the russets and golds of his garden. Some art historians, determined to look on the bright side, like to claim that his diminished sight opened up new spheres for him, a more inward vision that was dependent on knowledge and spiritual insight rather than direct perception. What is true is that he knew the colours of his garden at Giverny in a way that he could not have known those of any other landscape, since he himself had designed and supervised the construction of every path and bridge, planned the ponds, laid out the shapes of the flower beds, and directed the planting of all that was to grow therein. He worked in a hangar-like studio in a corner of his garden, choosing colours and forms dictated by his mind's eye while he painted the series for which he has become most famous, the enormous water-lily panels that were later installed according to his own directions in the Orangerie in Paris.

Monet once said he wasn't sure deep down whether he was actually more a gardener or a painter. Marcel Proust, who was an avid admirer of Monet's work, said that if one day he could see M. Claude Monet's garden he felt sure he would be looking at something that was not so much a natural flower garden as a colour garden, because it was planted in such a way that only the flowers with matching colours would bloom at the same time, harmonized in an infinite stretch of blue or pink. In those latter years the artist would have been able to see only the broad forms of his ponds and willow trees and bridges, and of the details not much at all, but it seems not to have mattered. <u>The artist, after all, strives not to imitate nature but to imitate its Creator,</u> and <u>art needs no reality beyond its own.</u> As Proust said, "*Le peintre traverse le miroir magique de la réalité.*"

I CHECKED around the dining room. With my new eye, the yellow wallpaper appeared to be brighter, clearer, but not altogether changed in character the way the blue was. The same for the coral-red seats of the chairs, which looked as though they'd had a good washing perhaps, but were not utterly different. It seemed that although blue had been forced to reveal itself in previously unimagined brilliance, red and yellow were still more or less able to take my new powers in stride. It had been a dull and rainy morning, but after a belated breakfast I noticed that the sun was coming out, so I walked into the living room and looked toward the large front window. In the sudden blast of light tears sprang and flooded my new and still photophobic eye, but through the mist I could see the fresh rosy brick of the house across the street, the sparkle of a bicycle anchored to its iron railings, the deep viridian leaves of the maple tree next door, the dazzling emerald of the vines around the windows. And the sky. <u>Oh my God, the blue sky!</u>

Helen McLean has followed a dual career as an artist and writer. She is the author of two novels, two memoirs, and a collection of essays. Her novel Significant Things *was shortlisted for the 2004 Commonwealth Writer's Prize, Canada/Caribbean division. Her paintings are in many private and public collections, including the Margaret Laurence Home in Neepawa, Manitoba, and the Bank of Canada, Ottawa. Recent articles, reviews, and essays have appeared in* The Globe and Mail, Brick, *the* National Post, Books in Canada, Literary Review of Canada, Quill & Quire, Room of One's Own, Ars Medica, *and* Accenti Magazine. *Her books include* Sketching From Memory: A Portrait of My Mother *(Oberon, 1994),* Of All the Summers *(Women's Press, 1999),* Details from a Larger Canvas *(Dundurn Press, 2001),* Significant Things: A Novel *(Dundurn Press, 2003), and* Just Looking and Other Essays *(Seraphim Editions, 2008).*

Lethargy, Resulting from the Sudden Extinction of Light

Mary O'Donoghue

Based on Jean-Martin Charcot's 1880s *Iconographie: Photographs of Patients with Hysteria, Salpêtrière Hospital, Paris*

The nurse looks away from the patient
whose back is arced in a swoon
in her arms, a skin and bone parabola.

She rolls her eyes to their corners
as if to say: I'm fed up with this
light–dark, fall–catch charade,

I'm sick of bracing my knees
in wait for the sudden drop
of their weight, I'm sick

of the smell of their blackouts,
sweat on serge or wool, sour
as ammonia. Their impromptu

urine, warmly worming down
my own skirt and over my shoes.
And I don't believe them anyhow.

Her hands are clasped against the patient's
ribs, thick washerwoman's fingers,
latticed like skin and bone basketwork.

She does not understand Doctor's modus
operandi, and why these women
faint away when the light is quenched

like a match disappeared into
a mouth. She lets their heads
loll back, inept new mother.

She holds her pose, a tedious pietà,
in the dark. She hears the glass of photo
plates slide like swords into a magician's box.

Swallows

The opening lines of this sestina come from Elizabeth Grey Countess of Kent's remedy for "Sinews That Are Shrunk," in *A Choice Manuall, or Rare and Select Secrets in Physick and Chryusurgery* (1653).

Take young Swallows out of the nest, a dozen or sixteen,
and Rosemary and Lavender, and rotten strawberry leaves . . .
afeer the quantity of the Swallows, the feathers, guts and all,
bray them in a mortar and fry them all together . . .
then put it in an earthen pot, and stop it close nine days . . .
when you shall use it chafe it against the fire.

She should call him in, push him towards the fire,
big bear of a boy in a yeti coat. He is sixteen
and standing on the lawn patchworked with leaves.
Sweet crumbs in his pockets from biscuits for all
the dogs on the road. Eyes too close together.
He likes outside when rain sedates the days.

Every June makes her think of other sizzling days,
sandals on tarmac as viscous as rubber from fire.
Walking the pram, she and her sister (sixteen,
fawn-legged, caramelized skin). Short shelter from leaves
of three larches. No sounds from the pram at all.
A baby with hands clasped watertightly together.

Her sister goes back to school, and they are together.
She waits and loses count of the days
of waiting for his eyes to spark, catch fire,
and swallow her face. Twelve months, sixteen,
then twenty, and nothing. Waiting. She leaves
it so late. A shocked doctor's questions, when all

she meant was to give him time. But all
the doctor sees is angry rash, toes webbed together.
Muscles slack as a rag doll's. Tests last for days
and she is sent home. She falls asleep by the fire
and dreams of feeding him, fleshing him. Sixteen
stone of him now kickwalks through wet leaves

towards the shed with the nest. He never leaves
little things to themselves, and crushed all
the baby swallows, trying to cup them together
in his red slabs of hands on one of the days
last week. She tipped open-beak chicks in the fire.
Fire-cracks from bones, pluck stench. He is only sixteen.

At thirty, his face is sixteen. He leaves for the home in October
with all of his clothes in two bags. White van doors smack together.
The days starve her down. Birds scream at her from the fire.

Mary O'Donoghue is an Irish poet and novelist. Her poetry collections are Tulle *(Salmon Poetry, 2001) and* Among These Winters *(Dedalus Press, 2007). Her novel* Before the House Burns *was published by Lilliput Press in 2010.*

On the Loss and Reconstruction of a Self

Menorah Lafayette-Lebovics Rotenberg

As I write this now in 2007, "I" am "myself" again. But where was my "self" and who was "I" for the most part of the year 2000–2001? In April 2000 I was diagnosed with both a lung disease, MAI (mycobacterial avian interstitial pneumonia, a disease akin to TB but not contagious) and with breast cancer. Following a lung operation (which provided the diagnosis) and a mastectomy (my second, the first was my fortieth birthday present), I was placed immediately on several strong antibiotics for the MAI, and soon after began chemotherapy for the cancer. These medications suppressed my appetite for food and altered my sense of taste in such a profound way that I no longer recognized myself. What does it mean to lose one's appetite? And how does that spread—like a cancer itself—to a loss of appetite for living? Coincidentally, at this time, Nitai, my two-year-old grandson's favourite words were "I want!" shouted with great expectation and glee, leading me to puzzle over what happened to my desire. Susan Sontag wrote her renowned *Illness as Metaphor* while recovering from cancer. Her ability to do this was a mystery to me. How did she manage it? How did she maintain her desire? I was in the middle of writing an article on the character of Rebecca in the Hebrew Bible that I had started earlier in the year. I could not continue to work on it. It felt foreign to me. I shrank into myself, not venturing out except to keep medical appointments. I, who loved to roam the streets of Manhattan, finding wonderful cafés like the light airy one at the Pierpont Morgan Library that was built around a large tree because they did not want to cut it down, now hated to run even a simple errand. I was losing the self I was used to and I missed it grievously.

I was reminded of myself when I was ten and my mother took me to see Stella Chess—who later was to become a pre-eminent child psychiatrist—to see if she could help rid me of my facial tics. It was as if she were a magician as she seemingly whisked away the grimaces—which were never to appear again. Where did they come from and where did they go? This "disappearing act" instilled in me a lifelong curiosity about the nature of consciousness, the connection of psyche and soma, and the nature of volition. I had tried so hard to get rid of the tics and suddenly they were effortlessly shed. It gave me a lasting respect for the formidable power of the unconscious, and an enormous belief in the transforming power of psychotherapy.

If tics disappear, we say goodbye and good riddance. But what do you say when you feel your very self is disappearing? How could I make sense of this? As a psychotherapist, I understood that our earliest self emerges, as Freud put it, from a body ego. We are embodied selves and we do best to remember that. Thus not only did I lose my appetite in general, but even when hunger (albeit in the guise of nausea) drove me to eat, I could no longer tolerate the foods I had always loved. Now it may be that there are many things that I don't know about myself. But going as far back as I can remember, one thing I always knew was that I had very definite tastes in food. I loved sweets and salty foods with a passion. My mother thought neither was healthful, so my grandmother, bless her soul, would let me have candy and soda on the sly. When I was eleven, one of my best friends and I would buy a bunch of radishes and take them to either her house or mine and sprinkle gobs of salt on them as our favourite snack. Now I could no longer tolerate sweet or salty foods and recoiled at the sight of my pantry stocked with bags of jelly beans, Reese's Pieces, M&Ms, pretzels, and potato chips. One of my favourite coffee spots in the Riverside Square Mall in Hackensack featured dense chocolate cake with Cointreau. I confess that at times I used to have that for lunch! I loved that mall, which I called "my mall" partly for its name, which reminded me of Riverside Drive in Manhattan where I spent a large part of my life. But I also loved it because there was an intimate feeling to it. There were always fresh flowers to lift my spirits, and in the winter the large skylight let in the bright warm sun and made it feel like an oasis in my hectic life. During my illness, however, it never beckoned to me. Indeed I never went out to eat because I was afraid that I would be unable to find on the menu the little I could tolerate. I was fast becoming a recluse overwhelmed by and preoccupied with my body. This preoccupation with my body could have become my new self, but I did not want to forge a new identity as a "sick person"—even though initially I resented all the healthy people around me. Some New Age cancer books spoke of the need to embrace one's illness. But I did not want its cold, unfeeling, dispassionate embrace. Intellectually I tried hard to distance myself from our Western dualistic notion of mind and body, but in my heart I wanted only to run away from my illness. The last thing I wanted was to embrace it. If I could have stayed out of my body until "it" got better, I would have done so. I was reminded of my fantasy during my first pregnancy when I wished I could unzip my uterus with my baby safely inside, put it aside while I ate and digested my food, and then zip it back in. Then too I wanted to escape from my body, from the constant indigestion that remained, even when the nausea abated. At that time we lived in Brookline, a suburb of Boston. There was a Howard Johnson's at Coolidge Corner where I took the train into Boston. They had banana flavoured ice cream, which I kept in the freezer. When I ate it I found relief and comfort, imagining that the cream was coating my stomach and warding off the acid causing the indigestion. But now food had become my enemy. I kept asking myself, "Who is this person who can no longer be comforted with ice cream?"

When I went to buy a wig, well-wishers told me that now I had the opportunity to reinvent myself. They suggested I experiment with a different style and colour. They meant to be helpful but they just did not understand. I did not want a new me, I wanted my old self back. I wanted to love listening to music again and to sing. I wanted to appreciate a beautiful day. I wanted to enjoy shopping again. I wanted to get back to writing. I wanted to get back to my ballet classes and enjoy the sheer animal pleasure of lithe movement. I loved my ballet classes. Even though I was by far the oldest in my class, being in my sixties, I shared a camaraderie with of all the young dedicated dancers, and our wonderful teacher. Of course it was hard for me to keep up—not easy to do sixty-four changements (jumps, with your toes pointed down switching left and right feet with each jump), at the end of class. Once I was lagging so far behind that my teacher Wendy said, "Menorah, the idea of jumping is that your feet leave the ground!" We all had a good laugh about that—and I desperately wanted those good times back!

But basically, I wanted to want. I missed my desire to desire. I wanted to be like my little grandson, Nitai, with his sweeping "I wants." I wanted to be comforted by enjoying the objects of my desire. Outings, family, and friends were immeasurably helpful and extraordinarily welcome. But I felt them only as a distraction, not as pleasure. I cut the tulips and lilacs and roses from my garden and dutifully put them into vases carefully positioned around the house, because my old self would have done so. The new, as yet un-named "me" was not moved by their beautiful subtle colorations, nor pleasured by their fragrance. We had a treasure trove of luscious raspberries in our backyard. Each year we shared our bounty with different friends and had an elegant "berry party." One year I asked my ten-year-old son, Ethan, "Whom should we invite over this year?" He replied, "No one, let's eat them all ourselves!" I loved his hearty unabashed greediness. Now, I pushed myself to gather the raspberries and to invite some friends over. While they enjoyed the scintillating fragrance and taste of the ripe just-picked berries, coupled as they were with heavy cream and sugar, and pastries, I toyed with the few berries I had put on my plate.

As I write this, I realize that my bewilderment and complaints sound like depression. Of course I was depressed. I was already seeing a therapist, but it was not helping and I stopped. All my neurotic issues paled before this megadose of physical reality. Nor did I think an anti-depressant would help something that was so physically and chemically based. I was pinning my hopes on my belief that when I accommodated to the medications, when I recovered from my three operations, when my hair grew back, and a certain amount of time would pass—with time itself being healing—I would begin to feel like my "sixty-three-year-old self." In that sense I would shed my depression as effortlessly as I had shed my tics sixty-three years ago.

As embodied selves we recognize that it is our senses that fuel our passions. When they are assaulted, we lose our very sense of ourselves. This is what often happens with aging. I remember being with my eighty-nine-year-old mother a few weeks before she died. She was very frail, could hardly stomach any food, and had trouble seeing. At one point she asked me, "Can you believe this is me?" and in truth I could not. What had turned this powerhouse of a woman into someone neither she nor I recognized? As one by one her senses failed her, she was becoming lost to herself.

What kind of a self do we construct as we become depleted selves? How does one agree to remain housed in a body poised to destroy one's self? If ever there was a "house divided against itself" threatening to bring down the entire partnership, this was it. And while we can attempt to mount a war against it, we cannot punish it, or bring it to justice. For this criminal who lurks in the shadows is in some inexplicable way also ourselves. "It" was indissoluble from my self. How do we begin to comprehend and make peace with this puzzle? How do we feel integrated and cohesive when faced with bodily disintegration? Do we ask too much of ourselves in thinking that we can maintain an integrated self? The thing about this puzzle, for me, is that even though this may place yet an additional burden on the ailing person, we long for that wholeness. For Jacques Lacan, the eminent French psychoanalyst, that constitutes the most early and basic denial. We do not want to accept that we are lacking and so as the two- (or three-) year-old looks into the mirror she constructs a unified image of herself. He suggests, it is that core cohesive image that flies in the face of reality that we always hanker for and are never able to attain.

The thing about adapting to bodily changes is that, even if they are pleasurable changes, it takes time to incorporate them into a body image. At age eighteen, I had my nose reshaped. I had been looking forward to it, I wanted it with all my heart, and I loved the way I looked afterwards. But it took me months of looking in the mirror to recognize and incorporate the new look as "me." Similarly, after my hair grew back, I decided not to colour my hair, as I loved the various shades of pearly white and grey. But for months I would catch a glimpse of my reflection walking by the windows of the stores in "my mall" (to which I had now, after a year, thankfully returned) and think, There's an interesting looking person who looks a little bit like me. Then I would realize it was me. But it took many months before that interesting looking person melded into myself.

Eventually, almost a year after I began treatments, I began to feel better and began to feel like my old self. It was an incremental process, thus quite the reverse of how it set in so precipitously. Slowly I accommodated to the medications and began to look forward to eating again. After a year of healthy food only because that was the only kind I could tolerate, I began to embrace junk food again. I went back to the café in "my mall" and savoured the anticipation of having that wonderful moist, chocolaty Cointreau cake for lunch that may have been bad for my body, but was like a wonderful restorative balm for my psyche. As I had lost ten pounds, I gleefully would ask for hot chocolate with whipped cream to have with it. In writing this, I continue to be puzzled and plagued with this psyche and soma dualism and do not know how to get around it. Yet while I am puzzled by it, I do know this: I have been restored to my old self by denying that my body will betray me yet again. In confronting my mortality, I lost myself. Who can desire, when death may be around the corner? Marcio De F. Giovannetti writes of "the pain associated with knowledge or the rejection of the knowledge as a result of which the human being discovers what constitutes both his greatness and his more drastic limitation—the erogenous and mortal body." In believing that, even if I am not cured, I hope to have many more years to live, I have been able to reclaim myself. I look different and I look older. But I am ready to have fun again. I am ready to embrace my grandson's credo of "I want!" Adam Phillips, who writes so masterfully about desire, writes that "children are, as their parents always say, impossible. They want more than they can have. And at least to begin with, they are shameless about it." It has taken me awhile, but I have my old self back: in my daily life and professional life I am Menorah Rotenberg again. With the name Menorah Lafayette-Lebovics Rotenberg I have resumed writing again—witness this essay—using my nom-de-plume. How I chose that name is a story in itself for another time.

References

Sontag, Susan. *Illness as Metaphor*. New York: Farrar, Straus and Giroux, 1978.

Lacan, J. *Écrits: A Selection*. London: Tavistock, 1977.

Giovannetti, Marcio De F. "The Scene and Its Reverse: Considerations on a Chain of Associations in Freud," in *A Child Is Being Beaten*, edited by Ethel Person, 95–111. New Haven: Yale University Press, 1997.

Phillips, Adam. *The Beast in the Nursery*. New York: Pantheon Books, 1998.

Menorah Lafayette-Lebovics Rotenberg is a psychotherapist in private practice. She writes primarily on the Hebrew Bible as viewed through the lens of a therapist. Her recent work on the matriarch Rebecca has appeared in Conservative Judaism.

The Cure of Metaphor

Kenneth Sherman

Heart
So there you are at last,
on the diagnostician's screen,
fluctuating between clinical grey
and amber, your chambers
opening and closing:
a mollusc
kneading its vital fluid.

You look so primitive.
Who would suspect you to inhabit
a human chest, to fasten
with such tenacity
onto a touch, lyrics,
frames of an old black
and white film?

Hoarder. I lie awake at night
hearing you thump thump
as if you were banging on the door
of my life, pleading
for one more chance
to wipe the slate clean
and begin again.

Venus Occluded

I awoke one morning to discover one eye
Weird, blurry, as if opened underwater.
At first I thought I was imagining the effect,
Denial my reaction to any physical mishap.
But two days later I found myself sitting
In the darkened chamber, the ophthalmologist
Hunched over me, his miner's light probing
The flooded landscape of my retina. "There it is."
Then the ominous pause. "A venous occlusion . . .
Some damage . . ." I understood occlusion as blockage,
But not being from the scientific side of things
Or wanting, perhaps, to accept responsibility for failed vision
I heard him speak the name of the goddess
And wondered if those images were fading
Because they'd not been loved enough.

Kenneth Sherman has published ten books, including The Well: New and Selected Poems *and* Void & Voice, *a collection of essays. His book-length poem,* Black River, *is forthcoming from Porcupine's Quill.*

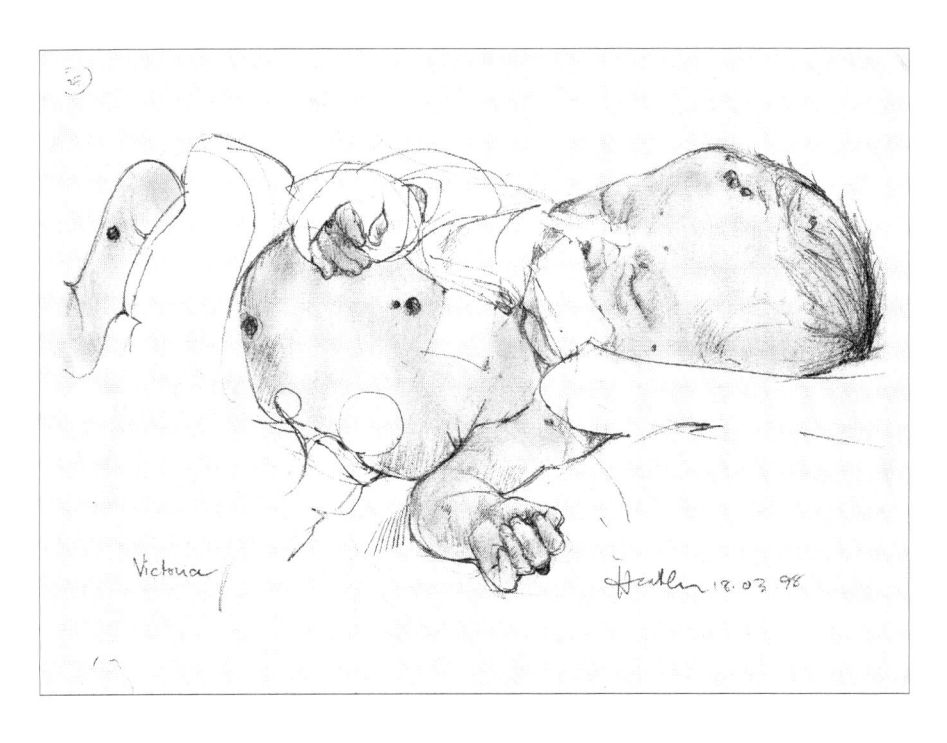

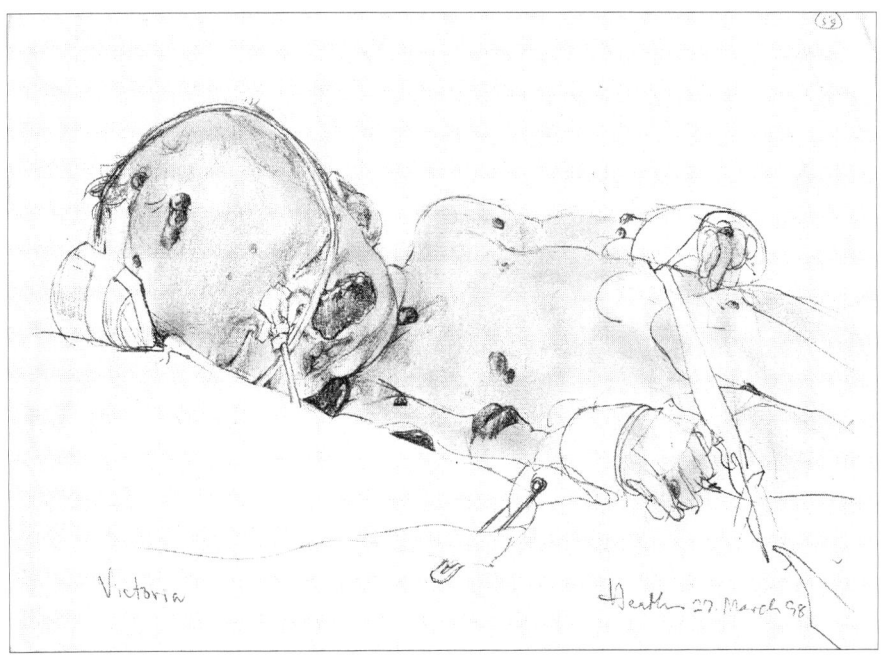

Drawings by Heather Spears

Kasabach-Merritt Syndrome

Heather Spears

The anticipated two-fold name
part-Prussian even, the stacked pages and graphs
are beyond me, the blackish photographs,
words like *hemangomia, vascular,*
primitive angioblast,
self-limiting, transient, cosmetic and benign
and then to scare me: *or*
morbid and cavernous.

I turn back to the table, the harsh light
where you lie without protest
naked, new born,
your skin is grey and ill
like fine sand weightless, weighed down
your life's violence and possibility
presenting only
in this scattering of dark lesions, visible and terrible.

Described as *warm to the touch,*
taut, pulsatile, without audible bruit.
A string of three across your brow
blood-red and shiny, so my pencil
leaps and cringes. More on your belly, your side,
while down your gauzy arm and at your throat
swarm the enlarged and involute:
black, foamy, petrified.

I draw a listless hand
finger by finger, the forgivable
minutiae of nail, knuckle, and on the third, there—
a berry, a sudden ruby!

Ruby. In a word I see you, the air
goes clear as water, you're
bejewelled then, bedecked as with coral
rising, its gems and encrustations
islands of breathing silence, you are star
studded, manifold, and my hand
steadies, my vision
writes indelibly, as with points of diamonds.

Heather Spears has published thirteen collections of poetry, four novels, and three books of drawings. Among her awards is the Governor-General's Award for Poetry.

Inadequacy of Impotence

George J. Stevenson

You flat-headed word.
You worm of a flat-headed word.
You wimp of understatement,
echo of *importance*. You imp,
you devil tormentor.
Im is close to *in*, yet *in*
is what you don't permit.

You sanitized word, hiding
in your medical guise.
Miscreant maladjusted
nothing word. Non-fucking
word with no clue
of how we live with you.

George J. Stevenson, diagnosed with prostate cancer in 2005, had radical prostatectomy surgery. He wrestled with the inability of mere words to express his feelings about the potential side effects of incontinence and impotence.

Diabetes:
My Body Says "Fall"

Heather L. Stuckey

Last night, I had a low blood sugar. Waking, confused, I called for Sue. Stumbling to find the low blood sugar machine, I turned on the closet light so as not to disturb anyone. My legs were weak, and I let myself fall to the floor. I checked my sugar, and it was 45. This is the number that makes my skin sweat like water drops and my body feel like clay. *Clay* is a good word, because my body becomes drenched like the consistency of it, solid underneath a sheath of salty water. It becomes mouldable and movable with pressure. My brain does not work, and so my body says fall.

Quickly, I drank six ounces of Hawaiian Punch, as if it were a secret potion. Life is fragile when Hawaiian Punch is the determining factor as to whether I live or die.

I gulp it and hear my heartbeat. Taking a deep breath, I realize my heart is louder than the volume of my inhalation. I wanted to capture each feeling, each sensation, so I could record what the experience of having a low blood sugar is like. I am trying, but it is coming out wrong. I am describing events, but not the actual feelings. If I were to ask you how to explain how it feels to touch a kitten or a pup, you might use words like *soft, cuddly, warm*, but it doesn't describe how your skin feels inside. What is the sensation, and how do you capture the experience of it?

Having a low blood sugar is like walking as a ghost through an imaginary, invisible world of the not-quite-dead and the not-quite-living. It is that space that hangs between hallucination and reality. I asked Sue where I was, and she said I was in my own bed. I tried to count backwards to make sure I was still on earth. Eight, ten, seven, six ... no, that wasn't quite right. Oh, God. I am losing my mind. What is the name of my son? Where do I work? I don't remember. I can't think. It has something to do with the letters *L* and *P*. Think. Think. I am cold.

Sue says I should lie down. I am catatonic, staring in space while holding a frantic discussion with myself. She takes off my sweat-filled nightshirt and dries my arms, my torso, my chest with a towel. She replaces a new nightgown and peels off my underwear like it is Saran Wrap. The sweat holds it in place and struggles against her tug. I am still raw and not strong enough to wait until she replaces my bedsheet with another towel. I have sweated the bed. I give up and fall to the floor. My forehead touches the ground and the bristles of the carpet feel like jagged glass. Everything is louder, more sensitive, on edge, too much. I have never had to take a psychedelic drug for this reason: it is enough to have a low blood sugar.

I feel the punch enter my bloodstream, warming and relaxing my body. It slows down my heart, allows me to return to earth. I still can't think clearly, but I know that I am on my way down. It is a trip back to reality, back to my bedroom. Soon I will sleep. It will be time for me to rest. The journey will have exhausted me. Vulnerable, yet safe, I close my eyes. I have lived through another night in the world of the near-dead.

Heather Stuckey, a D.Ed. candidate, has had Type 1 diabetes for twenty-five years and is involved in the Penn State Diabetes Center. She has a son, aged ten, and lives near Harrisburg, PA.

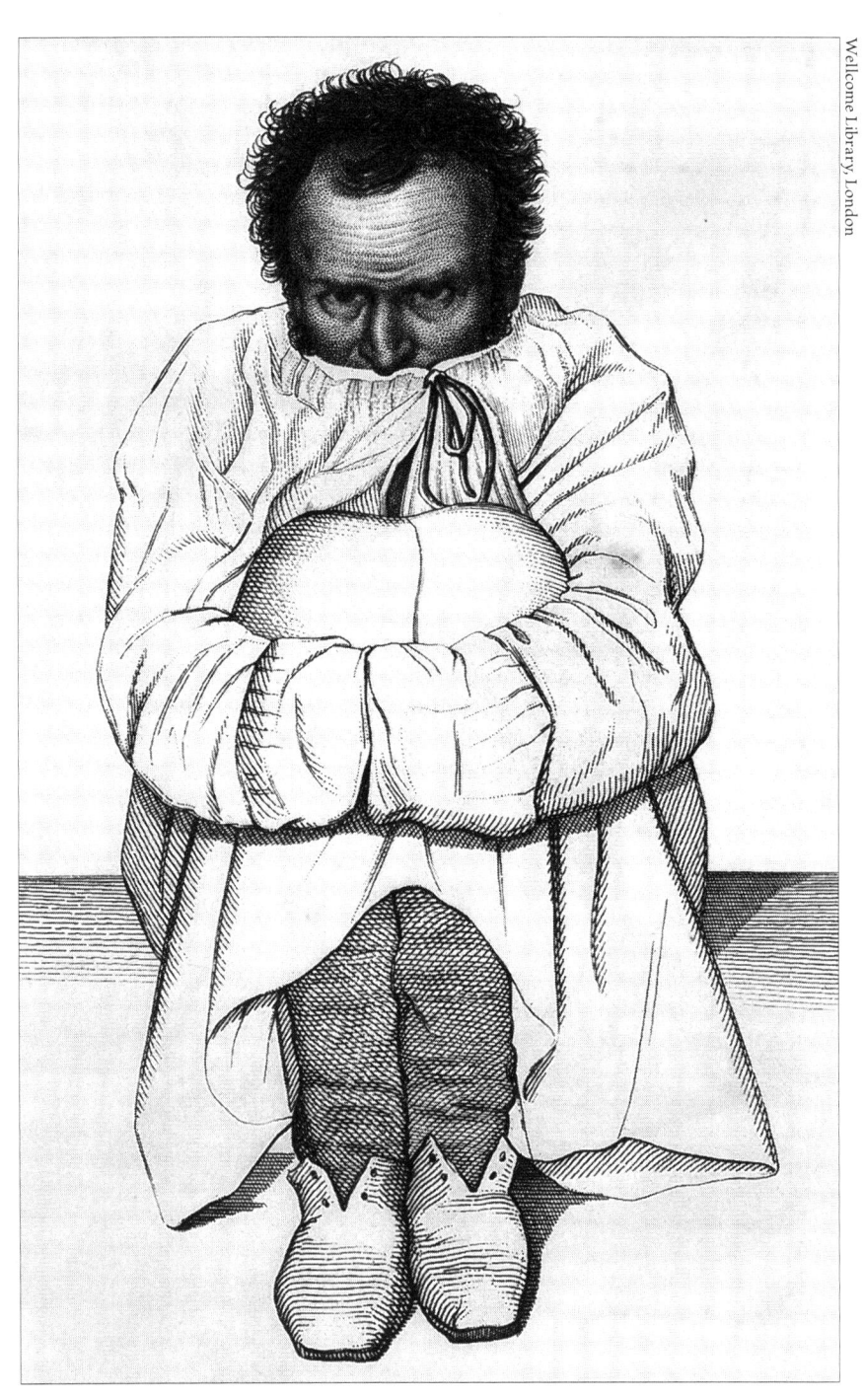

Ambroise Tardieu, "Mania Succeeded by Dementia," Des maladies mentales, *vol. 2, 1838*

Care for the Patient

Yvonne Trainer

In response to Ambroise Tardieu's engraving "Succeeded by Dementia"

He engraves each curl of his unwashed hair
with a swift sharp swirl
Engraves the curved lines of his forehead
In a few smooth cuts
chisels the dark and staring eyes
Engraves the cord that ties the robe
knowing I suppose the patient has forgotten
the usefulness of cords
Engraves the patient's shoes open without laces
so he will not fall
He does not draw the hands
hidden in sleeves of the robe
Hands that wrap
around the knees while the patient
stares and rocks stares and rocks
cold and afraid
afraid and cold.

Yvonne Trainer holds a PhD in contemporary literature (special topics area in medical humanities). She has published a chapbook and four books of poems and is an assistant professor at University College of the North.

I, Michael

Christopher Willard

Sheila's blonde hair catches the blue-white light scattered from the sheet of diamond-plastic covering the fluorescent lights. The strands spray glitter. Tinsel on a tree abandoned on a crisp winter's day. She bends toward me.

Sheila flies with the élan of a spring leaf.

Sheila parts her hair just left of the middle. When she looks down, her fine hair skims her high cheekbones and catches on her silver star-shaped earring. She raises her palm and dips her middle finger to slide the strand across her temple.

"Someday I will marry you, Michael."

She means me, I know. She means me in all my wan, penumbral, bedraggled form.

Sheila aligns her eyes with mine. I believe she seeks reassurance, a trait common with those who possess beauty.

"We'll have a big wedding and we'll fly to Rome on Air Italia. We'll visit the Vatican and the Campidoglio. We'll lay in the hot sun of the Borghese Gardens and we'll sip iced granita at a sidewalk café."

We both know she lies.

When it came time for Lodovico de Lionardo Buonarroti Simoni to name his son, he named him Michael. Michael the Angel. Inside a simple mayor's house wedged into the chestnut trees on a hill of Cabrese was born the greatest artist who ever lived. Michelangelo. That is how I would begin a book about him.

Michelangelo spent much of his early life reconciling a devotion to beauty against a failed piety. He wrote, "Already at age sixteen my mind was a battlefield: my love of pagan beauty, the male nude, at war with my religious faith." He personified his interior war by carving the twisted mass of human flesh he imagined in the battle between the Lapithae and the Centaurs.

When he was twenty-one he gave up routine depiction. While other artists sought the exterior model, Michelangelo strived for beauty that flowed directly from the hand of the divine, just as life flowed to Adam through the fingertip. He carved a standing Bacchus. Bundles of Sangiovese grapes form the ringlets of Bacchus's hair. He leans on a young satyr who stuffs a similar bunch of the sweet morsels into a laughing mouth. The youthful zymologist holds a cylix of wine that must contain a quart and a half. Art historians define his tilted stance as *contrapposto*. I think he's just half drunk. I know that legal drinking age in Italy is sixteen. Sometimes I imagine myself holding a cylix of wine filled with a Chianti or Merlot. In my imagination I stand in a similar pose, one knee slightly bent, hip and shoulder thrust toward each other, a posture of bravado and youth.

I've known Sheila for more than a year and I consider her my girlfriend. When I first confided this to her, she laughed the way a tree might laugh in the path of an avalanche, with unmoving knowledge of the inevitable. When I tell her now, she giggles with the litheness of a sparrow hopping along a wire. I may not say so directly, but I am in love with her and she is in love with me.

Sheila enters the room and leans toward me. I feel her long fingers smoothe my forehead and I think that she will marry me.

Some day.

Her eyebrows arch and she smiles as though she can read my thoughts. Or she smiles because she smiles. In all the time I've known her I've never seen her not smiling.

How long has Sheila been my ideal? She is the girl in every book. She is the girl pumping on the swing, the girl sleeping under the tree, the girl waving from a distance. Yet, oddly enough, I never dreamt about her. I don't dream of her now.

At ten years of age children slap snowballs against garage doors. Double that time and Michelangelo hammered his chisel into virgin marble alongside the greatest sculptors in the world. The innocence of his childhood somehow disappeared during those critical ten years. In a few days I will turn twenty-three. When Michelangelo was twenty-three his calipers first spanned the stone that would become the *Pietà*. It is the age when Michelangelo grew from boy to man, from a carver to a caresser. Not long after the *Pietà* was placed in St. Peter's Basilica, Michelangelo overheard a viewer credit Cristoforo Solari for the sculpture. I remember looking up Solari's work—I found it flat, dull, devoid of volume. Contrast this with the serpentine poses of Michelangelo's sculptures that breathe with a taut, bulbous life. Michelangelo returned to the Basilica and carved MICHEL ANGELUS BONAROTUS FLORENT FACIBAT, 'Michelangelo Buonarroti made this,' across Mary's sash. It is said to be the only work he ever signed. They say if Mary were to stand up, she would stand over ten feet tall. But she too is the ideal, and why shouldn't she be larger than life?

Sheila reads from Giorgio Vasari's *Lives of the Artists*: "It would be impossible to find a body showing greater mastery of art and possessing more beautiful members, or a nude with more detail in the muscles, veins, and nerves stretched over their framework of bones, or a more deathly corpse."

I lie staring at the ceiling, cherishing her throaty whispers and revelling in the airy scent of the perfume she touches to the back of her neck. Finally, she places a strand of hair between the pages and says she must go. I tease her and say I am in love with a woman who never has enough time for me. She cries it isn't true, that she has as much time for me as I could ever want. I remind her that when we are married we will have all the time in the universe. Clocks will run backwards, we'll grow younger, we'll decline from looking in mirrors.

When I'm alone I have the time to consider her name. I am the "he" hidden in Sheila. I am the "i" that follows the "She." Sheila's name is two and a half syllables long. She's not quite "She-la" not quite "She-i-la." To say "She-la" does not linger and "She-il-a" is just congestive and vulgar.

I know three o'clock arrives because Sheila walks into the room. Her step is light, cushioned, the tap of a kitten's paw as it jumps onto a linoleum floor.

I move my mouth, "I knew you'd return."

"How could I ever forget you?"

She opens the curtain to invite the hot spring light. Her palm brushes a flush warmth across my cheeks.

"You're the sweetest," I mouth.

How many artists have their most famous work located on a ceiling? Michelangelo painted thirty-three panels onto the ceiling of the Sistine Chapel, a number one less than his age when he began the massive frescos. When Pope Julius II asked Michelangelo to paint the ceiling, the artist replied he was a sculptor, not a painter. The pope responded that it was a demand, not a question. Michelangelo worked steadily, creating more than three hundred figures. His beard became matted with paint, he paused only when exhausted, he slept with his boots on. He stood bent, backwards, in a painful contorted posture. Michelangelo wrote in one of his sonnets, "I seem a bat upon its back."

"Am I a bat upon my back?" I ask Sheila.

She pauses from her reading and presses her ring finger to mark the last whispered word. She refuses a response. She looks upwards and across my patchwork ceiling where reproductions of Michelangelo's works are taped. The central piece is a 12 x 9 reproduction of the Sistine Chapel ceiling, pre-restoration, from a Singapore printing company. Most are postcards. Some arrived from Vatican City bearing stamps that depict a smiling silver-toned pope, a slightly overexposed basilica under a screaming cyan sky, or a slender green and red capped woodpecker. A particularly oily and tattered card stamped "Roma" in bold red letters provides a faded panorama of the Palazzo Nuova. Another card details the model of the wooden crate-like wagon used to transport Michelangelo's David from the piazza della Signoria to the Academia. The 12,000 square feet of the Sistine ceiling required four years of nearly continual work. It took me less than one year of sporadic work to cover half of the 144 square feet comprising the ceiling of my room.

When a new postcard arrives, Sheila retrieves a tall wooden stool.

Michelangelo's works ascend to a heavenly sixty-five feet off the floor. Mine are pasted twelve feet high. When Sheila tiptoes upward to affix the print, I examine her rubber-soled sneakers and count the butterflies that float across her socks. Someone once sent me a 1,000-piece jigsaw of the Sistine Chapel ceiling. I asked Sheila if she wanted the puzzle but she said she prefers answers.

"Which Michelangelo work looks most like me?" Sheila asks.

I roll my eyes. I scrutinize the images above me. Can one ideal represent another ideal?

For Michelangelo his figures were examples of ideal beauty rather than simple representations. I think this is why so many of his sculptures are pupil-less, with white marble moons gazing inward. Michelangelo knew there was always more destiny in the unseen than in the seen. While Raphael strutted along the sun-drenched vias Michelangelo hunched his bent body from shadow to shadow into posterity.

And so I roll my eyes with the knowledge that Sheila's task is absurd. Still, I hold her image in my mind and I scan the pictures with the determination to apply this mental mirage. I observe the thin face of Eve, hidden behind God's shoulder as he reaches out toward Adam. I consider the Mary of the Florentine *Pietà* but quickly dismiss it because relating Sheila to an unfinished work is abhorrent.

"I cannot choose," I say.

Sheila accuses me. She says I mock her question. She turns down her lips, but eyes betray the facade the way crepuscular rays cut through storm clouds.

I don't tell her, but she is most like the Libyan Sibyl closest to the altar. I've known this for as long as I've known Sheila. The Sibyl has Sheila's thin nose, her small heavy eyelids, her rose petal lip, her subtle divining smile. A blush ribbon holds the Sibyl's golden braided hair, a flush of sunset fills her cheeks. She wears a dress of gold and violet, of knowledge and royalty. She sets down the book of prophecies. I point out the big toe that supports the serpentine body of the prophetess, without telling Sheila this is the figure I choose.

When I think of Michelangelo as a person I think of the way he depicted himself. It's there on the Last Judgment just to the right of centre. Saint Bartholomew holds a flayed skin painted in Michelangelo's image, with sagging form, hollow eyes, twisted head, a mouth stretched and vacant. Here was the man who attached a candle to his cardboard hat so he could work at night creating the most beautiful art in the world. Here was the man who could twist an iron ring door knocker as though it were made of lead. Was this how he perceived himself? He might have written, "What are the woes of flesh when confronted with divine beauty?" He might have, but that one is mine. When I look at the flayed image of Michelangelo I see a failing flesh enclosing a vibrant mind.

I see the present more than I see the future.

"What do you think?" I ask Sheila.

She looks beyond the book and through the window toward the darkening sky.

The big toe of Bacchus is bent, the first two toes of David are splayed. She knows I mean Babinski's sign. The big toe flexes upwards and the other toes splay outward when the bottom of the foot is stroked. It's a sign of spasticity, in my case an advancing paralysis caused by a lesion occurring between the brain and the lower spinal cord. I know it's probably a weakness to frame the world so personally. Sheila says she won't talk about such things.

Amyotrophic lateral sclerosis occurs most frequently in adults between the ages fifty-five and seventy-five, and they tell me it's extremely rare in someone as young as I am. Because of my age they try to be as non-invasive as possible, but at some point I'll get a tracheo and gastro tube in addition to my feeding tube. Twenty-five per cent of those diagnosed live more than five years. After reaching stage four, they live maybe a year. Michelangelo painted the Last Judgment at the age most people retire. He lived to be eighty-nine years old during a time when most people were lucky to reach fifty. I'll be lucky to reach twenty-five at a time most people near eighty-nine.

After painting the Sistine Chapel, Michelangelo wrote, "I felt as old and as weary as Jeremiah. I was only thirty-seven, yet friends did not recognize the old man I had become." He understood the limitations of a corporal vessel that never fulfilled its promise.

I ask Sheila who else she knows who has as many therapists as I do. I refer to the speech therapist, the swallowing therapist, and the physical therapist. Michelangelo wrote, "My feet unguided wander to and fro." Those are my feet too. How did the therapist put it? "Non-ambulatory functions, lack of purposeful movement." I tell Sheila I must be an actor since people are always considering my stages. And I think she must be smiling although her face is turned away from the bed.

Altogether Michelangelo spent ten years of his life in the Sistine Chapel accounting for about one-eighth of his life. If I live to be twenty-five I will have spent three years, or about one-seventh of my life, in this hospital room.

If I had to be any Michelangelo work I would be the Atlas Slave who bends under the weight of physicality. It's one of his late, unfinished sculptures. Michelangelo believed that once the physical matter was removed, the form, the soul, could be revealed. One art historian wrote that the unfinished state suggested the drama of the soul imprisoned by the body.

Sheila sets the book on the table and squeezes my limp hand. She adjusts the bright yellow BiPap tube and makes sure my covers are tucked. Michelangelo wrote, "If one destiny is equal for two lovers..."

Eventually the day will come when Sheila and I fly to Rome. We'll walk through Bernini's colonnade and across the square of St. Peter's. We'll discover the chapel and we'll cross the Alessandrinum mosaic floor. We'll stand on the swirling circles that represent life and we'll arch our backs and peer upwards toward the Creation.

But this image is too maudlin.

If I know Sheila, I know that when it happens it will remain the miracle of the commonplace, without a last judgment, without pigmented pomp.

She leans her head close to mine. In her eyes I can see the silvers and greens of a bright March day. I see the shining reflections caused by a thundershower. I see the unadorned simplicity of Sheila's sneakers slapping a sunburst of droplets from the puddles as she runs down the slick street.

Christopher Willard is a Calgary-based writer, visual artist, and teacher. His novel Garbage Head *(Vehicule/Esplanade, 2005) was shortlisted for three awards across Canada.*

Part 2: Friends and Family

Introduction

This anthology provides space for stories seldom told. Health care practitioners—part of the educated elite—have periodically written of their experiences, if (until recently) impersonally. More rarely, patients have told their tales in print. And the popular entertainment and news media are never loathe to tell a medical story. But, despite this attention, the family and friends of the patient (and the clinician) are most glaringly absent or, at best, given a stereotypical walk-on part. The worried sister, fingers to mouth. The angry parent or spouse, obstructing care. The misunderstanding, neglected spouse of the dedicated healer.

At a recent meeting of parents of children with a chronic illness the participants were asked if they had ever been offered the chance to talk about the experience of having an ill child. Less than half the hands went up. Had their children had ever been asked if they wanted to talk about their experience? Well under half. Had anyone ever asked if the child's siblings, friends, or other relatives wanted to talk? Not a hand was raised.

The family and friends rarely even penetrate the circle of care existing between health care practitioner and patient. In medical charts they may appear in a brief line describing the "social" situation of a newly admitted patient: "lives with wife," "lives on her own, daughter visits." They may re-surface in the "discharge plans." At times, in the presence of a vague or elusive patient, they may be called upon to provide "collateral history."

And yet the family and friends hold a unique position in the health care system, sharing the roles of both other central parties. Much of the care for the acutely and chronically ill falls, inevitably, to the family and, at times, the friends. The dedicated physician who sees her elderly patient for a half hour a month still leaves the other 42,170 minutes in the hands of others. And, as our population ages and health care services are reduced, the portion of care off-loaded to this group will increase dramatically.

Yet the family and friends are also, in important ways, like the patients they care for and love. A mother's illness becomes the daughter's; a child's cancer invades the father; a friend's grief becomes my own. The impact of illness on the family and friends is unique, important, and deserves attention, to the betterment of us all.

Rex Kay, MD

Drawing Insulin

Anonymous

The green numbers on the microwave tell me it is 8:45 p.m., time to administer insulin to my son. From the stainless steel soap dispenser beside the kitchen sink, I pump a generous blob of liquid soap onto my hands. I rub my hands together, interlocking my fingers; the soap bubbles emerge and rise between my fingers. I move my hands under the tap. The warm water cascades over them, taking the soap with it down the drain. I turn to dry my hands on the hand towel that hangs from the handle of the oven door. While I wonder when the hand towel was last changed, I do nothing about it. My hands and nails are so dry; the hand lotion applied several times a day has been wasted effort.

Type 1 diabetes was diagnosed on his sister's seventh birthday, mere weeks before his eleventh. His initial reaction was anger rooted in fear. "I'd rather die than have diabetes!" Mine was resignation. For three weeks there'd been the quenchless thirst, the bedwetting, and the trips to the bathroom in the middle of the night—symptoms recalled from television ads years before. I knew what was coming before the pediatrician confirmed it. And then, days at the hospital for diabetes day care: meetings with doctors, nurses, dieticians, and social workers; reams of information extracted from and thrown at us—checking glucose levels (highs, lows, and target ranges); counting carbs; measuring and administering insulin; managing illness; testing urine for ketones; the nightmare scenario that calls for glugacon. The unspoken mantra: Managing diabetes is about precision and routine, routine, routine. But life with a child, with my child, is never routine.

The glass vial with the orange ring around the top sits on the black granite counter. I pick it up and roll it gently between my palms as if I am rolling Plasticine. The contents turn cloudy as the white liquid settled at the bottom mixes with the clear liquid at the top. I return the vial to the counter and take a syringe out of the cardboard box beside the cookie jar. The side of the syringe is marked in millilitres, like the markings on a measuring cup. I remove the white plastic cap from the plunger end of the syringe and pull the plunger back and forth several times, taking care not to pull it out entirely. It glides smoothly. I remove the orange plastic cap from the needle end of the syringe and slowly pull the plunger back until the black top of the plunger inside the syringe is lined up perfectly with the eight-millilitre marking. White, orange and black—Halloween colours. This procedure has become so routine, the temptation to give in to distraction is powerful. But distraction equals mistakes: incorrect doses, midnight telephone consultations with residents on call, embarrassment coupled with a vow to myself never to repeat the error, and the knowledge I can't be certain I won't. How is it possible that some nights I lie in bed wondering whether I administered insulin to my beloved son? It has become too automatic—mere white noise in our lives.

How far we've come from those first few days when, observed by a nurse, it took two of us to restrain our flailing, screaming son just to administer a needle. Embarrassed that I'd raised such an angry, non-compliant child and dreading the prospect of our future battles, I blinked away tears and swallowed the rising lump in my throat. Two years on, he is resigned to his fate, though he evidences little interest in managing it himself. He tests his blood sugar on autopilot—the finger prick, drop of blood, and beep from the meter are prerequisites to the injection but he doesn't look at the reading; the purpose doesn't register—it's just something he has to do. Medicalert bracelets are purchased, donned, removed, and invariably lost. "It's stupid. I don't care!" He's not embarrassed about diabetes; he's pleased at an opportunity to share that information, but with little appreciation for all it entails. He accepts his three daily injections, but needles for any other purpose continue to terrify. My son who has endured more than a thousand injections, simply refused to join his classmates in the school-administered hepatitis vaccine and bridled for days at the prospect of a flu shot. "I hate needles. They hurt!" "Why do I have to have a flu shot?" "I don't want one and don't need one." And so it went.

And so it goes too. "Don't hurt me, Mommy," has become part of his routine, words spoken without thought, involuntarily I believe. Words I desperately try to ignore. I am tired—tired of inflicting the pain he cannot live without, tired of feeling that while much responsibility rests on me, I am no better than an adequate participant. Why don't I push him to take ownership of his treatment? He can self-administer but would rather not and, when pushed, seems nonchalant, even cavalier about it. And so, it is easier to do than to delegate and worry. Intellectually I know I am doing neither of us any favours. But I can't let go—not yet. He needs me, doesn't he?

Without moving the plunger, I insert the needle end of the syringe into the middle of the white rubber top of the vial and depress the plunger, pushing eight millilitres of air into the vial. I turn the vial upside down, placing the neck of the vial in the vee formed at the base of the forefinger and middle finger of my left hand so that my fingers alone support the vial. The syringe does not fall out. I form a circle, like an "OK" sign, with my right forefinger and thumb and, using that thumb for resistance, rapidly unfold the forefinger several times so it flicks out and hits the vial. A small air bubble is released from the neck of the vial and rises to the surface. I put my left thumb and baby finger on either side of the syringe to support it and use my right thumb and forefinger to pull the plunger down, drawing thirteen millilitres of insulin. I rapidly push the plunger back into the syringe so that all of the insulin is returned to the vial. I listen for a click and am rewarded. Air. Again, I draw, this time taking fourteen millilitres of insulin, and rapidly push the plunger, returning the insulin to the vial. No click this time. Using my right thumb and forefinger for control, I slowly pull back the plunger until its black top inside the syringe meets the eight-millilitre marking.

My days are filled with repetition—hundreds of little tasks, hundreds of thankless endeavours. I hold the syringe up to the light, looking for air bubbles, but find none. I carefully remove the syringe from the vial and call my son.

The author is the mother of three children living in Toronto. To preserve the family's privacy and her son's dignity she has chosen to publish in Ars Medica *anonymously.*

Days and Nights in NICU

Christine Benvenuto

My daughter was perfect. Thanks to a short suspension in the birth canal, she didn't have the battered prizefighter look that my first two children wore into the world. Okay, she was an amazing dark brick red but—as I would soon be told by an array of wannabe medical comedians—red was better than blue.

Born at thirty-six weeks, six days, the baby was a day shy of being considered full term. Clogged with amniotic gunk, in her first moments of life she spluttered and fussed instead of issuing the lusty newborn cries I'd heard twice before. The nurses cleared her nose with their powder blue plastic bulbs. When they took her off for her bath, I showered and moved into a postpartum room, then went to the nursery to claim my daughter. Nurses stood on either side of the bassinet, exclaiming to each other over her beauty. They had examined my baby and pronounced her healthy.

We spent our first night together in the postpartum bed. I gazed. She nursed, a little inexpertly. It was our honeymoon. In the morning she cried whenever I tried to put her down and made it clear that life had better arrange itself to keep her in my arms.

We planned to go home as soon as our pediatrician examined her, a formality. When the doctor arrived, around noon, they took the baby to the nursery. That's when it all began.

My husband was teaching that afternoon and had our three-year-old daughter with him. Our nine-year-old son, in love with his newest sister, elected to spend the day with the baby and me. So he was with me when I walked into the nursery to see how things were going. Once again the baby was in the bassinet, flanked by nurses. But now no one was smiling.

"She was breathing very rapidly," announced our pediatrician. Had I noticed a problem? I hadn't. The baby was hooked up to heart and respiration monitors, with her head under what looked like a clear plastic cake dome, an oxygen-enriched environment. In the minutes she'd been away from me, my daughter had entered the grip of medical crisis.

"Is this bad?" my son asked. Later he'd insist that the hospital couldn't hold his sister and threaten to notify the police.

I brought my son to my room and went back to the nursery. This was a path I'd retrace many times in the coming hours. Going to the nursery to be with my baby. Feeling in the way and concerned about leaving my son alone with his fears, returning to my room to be with him. Terrified of what might be happening, hurrying back to the nursery. One return, the doctor said the baby's eye movements might indicate seizure activity. I disagreed—I'd seen these twitching eyelids on dreaming babies before—but didn't say so, since my opinion would only be chalked up to denial. Later on, I was in my room for a moment while my husband, son, and daughter went to get some dinner. My son came in alone. Someone in the nursery had just told his father that the baby had an irregular heart beat. What, he wanted to know, did this mean?

My husband confirmed that the monitors had picked up a heart fluctuation. Coming on top of the rapid breathing and possibility of seizure activity, this was the low-tech nursery's last straw: the baby was being moved to the Neonatal Intensive Care Unit (NICU) of a much larger teaching hospital half an hour's drive away.

We threw ourselves into a numb flurry of activity. I cleared away the gluey remains of my children's pizza dinner. My husband made phone calls in search of someone to take the children for the night. I began losing things: the address book I'd been holding, then the baby's name. The name, just like the baby, was slipping through my fingers. In the midst of this, the midwife on duty sat down beside me on my hospital bed. "Do you think there is any way that this baby can be okay?" I demanded. She said, "Yes." What else could she say? Then she volunteered to bring our children to the friends' home where they would spend the night, and gave them the ride of their young lives in her jazzy top-down convertible.

After they'd left, someone remembered that I had given birth less than twenty-four hours before, and I realized that I was dizzy. A chair was brought to the foot of the bassinet, and I was given some sweet grape juice to drink that made me feel worse than I had before. My husband and I cooed to the baby and stroked her. She screamed at the top of her lungs, still brick red ("Better red than blue!") and unable to nurse with her head inside the oxygen dome.

The medical team that arrived from the teaching hospital were so green, the young intern insisted up front that he was a doctor, expecting to be contradicted. They gave the baby a dose of phenobarbital so that, if there had been seizure activity, it would be controlled during transit. They transferred her to an aptly named isolette, a clear plastic box on wheels, and she was on her way. We followed the ambulance in our own car, barely able to speak to each other.

We entered the NICU that night and over the coming days through a series of hurdles. The receptionist checked with a nurse to see if she could buzz us in. We performed the timed, two-minute hand scrub. Then we staggered through a dimly lit ward of bassinets and isolettes.

We found our baby in the last bassinet at the end of a row. There had been another moment of heart fluctuation upon arrival. Now she was resting. Oxygen was being pumped into her nose, an invasive procedure that we were told is sometimes effective at jump-starting newborn lungs. She was wired everywhere, bruises flowering where IVs lodged, needles jabbed, and tape attached things to her diaphanous skin, receiving antibiotics to treat an infection that might be lurking unseen, and sugared water since she couldn't nurse while on oxygen. But the rest of that night was quiet. In the morning they talked about letting her breathe on her own. When I heard that I would be able to nurse her again, I burst into pent-up tears.

She was put through a battery of tests: EKG, EEG, CAT scan, MRI, MRV, repeated blood tests, examinations by pediatricians, a pediatric neurologist, a geneticist. A spinal tap, excruciatingly painful even for adults, was performed twice before enough spinal fluid was collected.

We weren't allowed to be with the baby during most of these procedures. Because we'd arrived when one of the NICU's two family rooms was unoccupied, we had somewhere else to go. In this invaluable pocket of space—the sofabed, if unfolded, filled it—with its own bathroom we could take showers, and I could use the industrial-strength breast pump a nurse helpfully provided. We could rest, after a fashion. If we dozed off for a moment, the ringing telephone tore through our half-sleep, terrifying even though it was only a summons to nurse the baby.

We held her as much as possible, negotiating the mess of wires. She nursed, slept in our laps, or looked into our eyes, sucking on our fingers and fluttering starfish hands with graceful underwater movements. While she slept I read a long novel by Trollope, soothed by the characters' quiet, nineteenth-century self-destruction. Days slid into nights. The world outside the NICU windows seemed uniformly remote and grey. Parents came and went. We stayed. Across the aisle, a teenaged dad kept his own vigil beside his son's isolette.

Most of the NICU parents were teens or not much older, the very young parents of children with intricate needs. One day we overheard a nurse detail a baby's arsenal of medications to a young woman with limited English who would soon have to give them to her son at home; the tiny patient, about the same size as our daughter, was 100 days old. All the babies looked like newborns; many were weeks, if not months old. The isolets housed some of the tiniest human beings in existence. Like parents everywhere, we knew our daughter's cry. We also recognized the baby who bleated like a lamb, the one who mewled like a cat in trouble. But most of the babies made themselves known only through the warning beeps of their monitors.

The babies were assigned a nurse every twelve-hour shift. The majority of the nurses were smart and dedicated; a few looked to be passing the hours until the shift would end. The doctors comprised a uniformly brisk, businesslike group. That is, all except the young intern who had come to get our baby from the hospital where she was born. "He only knows what I tell him," one nurse told another. He tried to imitate the professional veneer of his older colleagues, hopelessly unable to carry it off. One day he wanted to tell me what an MRI was, and was clearly stumped. I explained it to him instead. "That's it!" he beamed, his inner incoherence mapped for him. The boy doctor provided us with our only moments of hospital humour.

People incidental to our baby's care were uncommonly kind: the maintenance workers who cleaned the family room and brought us fresh towels; the receptionist who allowed us to hang onto the room when the baby's discharge kept being delayed; the cafeteria cashier who asked after her every day, and stopped charging us for our purchases when she decided we'd spent enough; the diners who brought my purse to the cash register for safekeeping when I walked out of the cafeteria without it; and the social worker from another part of the hospital who visited because she knew us slightly, bringing compassion and a whiff of the outside world into our vacuum of crisis.

Throughout these days my husband shuttled back and forth between the hospital and home, an hour away, where our son and daughter were being looked after by his mother. Each day the kids came to the hospital to have dinner in the cafeteria. Each evening we faced the wretched moment of separation. My husband and son and I were stoically miserable. My daughter cried. Once, saying goodbye in the lobby, we saw a new mother leaving the hospital's childbirth facility with her infant, baby balloons flying. That's the way it's supposed to be, we told each other.

Sometimes one of our baby's alarms would go off, but these always turned out to be mechanical glitches. Our hearts would stop, but hers never again missed a beat. The pediatric neurologist saw no indication that she'd had seizures, and each test yielded normal results. Tubes and wires were removed, our baby was returned to us by degrees. Raw fear turned to a desperate impatience to get her home before they found an excuse to keep her.

But getting out of the NICU proved more difficult than getting in. Some of the tests had to be redone, either because they hadn't been done properly the first time or because their results were inconclusive. While some provided quick information, on others we had to wait for a few of our baby's cells to grow in a laboratory into health or abnormality. Considered premature, she had to pass a road test, proving that she could sit strapped into a car seat for sixty minutes while the oxygen absorbed into her blood stream stayed above 95 per cent. If it dropped—and it did, over and over—she couldn't go home. After trying out seat after seat, we finally understood that our daughter could ride home in a car bed, oxygen-rich and prone, anytime. In exchange for our credit card number, the bed was delivered to the NICU by a respiratory equipment company. I thought I was dreaming when the release forms were signed and handed over. I dressed the baby in the clothes her brother and sister had worn for their entrances to the world.

Before my daughter was born I believed I knew only one NICU alum. In fact I knew several. Not surprising, given that some 9 per cent of babies spend time in a NICU. As one mother said, people try to put the NICU behind them. They don't talk about it, while the trauma of the experience continues to haunt long after. In our family, from time to time a memory is triggered out of nowhere, and together we find ourselves reliving that painful week and its blessed outcome. We'll never know whether our baby's time in the NICU was beneficial, even necessary. For this we can only count ourselves lucky.

That last morning, when we were finally ready to go, there wasn't a single nurse or doctor in sight. We gathered up our baby and, with no one to say goodbye to, walked out of the NICU. We rode the elevator to the lobby. The hospital doors slid open and I carried my week-old daughter out into the sunlight for the first time.

Christine Benvenuto is the author of Shiksa: The Gentile Woman in the Jewish World, *published by St. Martin's Press, and her fiction and essays have appeared in many publications.*

Eden and I Are Playing Go Fish

Susie Berg

She wears a pink cap to cover her bald head.
She misses her hair.
A lot.
She's five.
There's a tumour on her brain.

Do you have any . . .

She stops
and studies her cards,
points one by one, silently counting spades.

. . . sixes?

Her mother shakes with laughter,
soundlessly,
clears away tears, touches
Eden's chin.

You make me so very happy.

Susie Petersiel Berg is a Toronto writer and mother of two whose work has appeared in several publications. Her chapbook of collected poems, Paper Cuts, *was published in 2007.*

Palliation

Pat Cason

My brother called me out of the blue. He'd always favoured the element of surprise. "Apparently I'm kicking the bucket," he said.

"Who is this?" I said. I was still a little mad. He'd blackmailed our parents, refused my phone calls, stamped *return to sender* on my letters. Not to mention the bicycle, the cat, the black paint. Now he was dying. You see my point.

I relented. "What was your first clue? You've been trying to kill yourself for years." That bucket he said he was kicking—I was curious to know if he really meant it, this time.

He did. "It's called palliative care. There's nothing else they can do. They just give me morphine for the pain"—this was back before the fancy anti-retroviral cocktails they give people now—"and even the morphine's not working so hot anymore. Although being under the influence is probably why I called you."

"I was wondering," I said, although I figured he just wanted to re-engage an audience he could then ignore, "I was wondering why you called, after refusing the letters I wrote."

"I steamed them open first, though," he said.

"You could've just written *fuck you* on the envelopes and sent them back."

"I considered it," he said, "but I didn't think the post office honoured requests like that."

WHICH IS ALL BY WAY of explaining why I flew to California to visit my nearly dead, only living relative.

"You must be the boyfriend *du jour*," I told the man with greying ponytail who answered the door. "I'm the sister from hell."

"Pleased to finally meet you," he enthused. "I'm Kip." He grabbed my hand and shook it with a fervour I found excessive.

"You don't fool me for a minute," I said. "Where's His Royal Highness?"

Smile gone, he motioned to the back porch.

My brother was stretched out on a chaise longue, eyes closed. Lifelike garden art: Gargoyle at Rest. I assumed he was rehearsing his death, or skipping out when things heated up, skills he'd perfected. Sunlit batik awnings splattered colour across him. It was an arboretum out there. I tried to ignore the begonias, reminded myself why I'd come. Reminded myself of the stop sign, the lawyer, the rotten peaches. Of the venom that kept us alive. Although now it felt like a toxin I had to flush out of my system, in order to live.

"Awful cheerful place to die," I said.

He opened one eye. "You have no idea."

"You're all sticks and bones." I sat on the chaise beside his.

"Men used to follow me home," he said, haughty. "They lined up at my door."

"You were buff," I agreed. "Look where it got you."

"And you," he said, "where did life get you?" He had a point.

"What's with the Cheerios?" A shelf held potted blossoms. Someone had scattered cereal O's across it, a surface printed as though by the random hands of tiny children.

He closed his eye. "Raccoons," he said, "maybe skunks. They come at night."

"Quite the nightlife you've got these days," I said, "feeding feral phantoms in the dark."

He ignored me, or didn't hear, because pretty soon I heard his quiet snoring.

A THUD, A CRASH, A MOAN. My brother didn't move. Inside the house I found Chip on the floor, clutching his chest, hyperventilating. He'd pulled down a bookcase. He was flailing a bit.

"You a drama queen too, or just a clumsy choreographer?" I helped him stand. "Your face is kind of grey, Skippy. Take a load off. I'll call 911."

He sank onto the bed and waggled a hand. "Heart condition," he said. "Ran out of nitro. May be fatal this time . . ."

"You ought to make an effort to speak in complete sentences," I told him, relying on the benefits of distracting the wounded from their pain.

He rolled his eyes. Drama queen, I decided. "If you're dying, just don't upstage him," I said. "He'd never forgive you."

WE WAITED for paramedics. Two strapping young men in good haircuts and pressed uniforms carried a collapsible gurney up the front steps. "If they're gay I'll slit my wrists," I told Pip. He smirked. Maybe he thought I was joking; I've carved myself for less. Must be zoning law, or a law of nature that every non-visitor within a mile of the Russian River at Monte Rio be gay. Too bad. I'll admit to lust as I watched from the window. Men in uniforms.

I let them in. "I gave him an aspirin," I said. "He thinks he's having a heart attack."

One of them took Mister Boyfriend's pulse and put a blood pressure cuff on his arm and clipped something to his finger. EMT Number Two fitted a plastic mask over his face, all business until he noticed a sheet of orange paper taped to the wall over the bed.

"Lookit this." He knuckle-thunked the paper.

They started unhooking things. "Hey," Boyfriend Guy muttered.

"Why'd you call us?" one of them asked me. "This says *Do Not Resuscitate*. It's legally binding. We can't take him anywhere."

"Check his ID," I said. "This isn't the nearly dead guy. Although he will be soon, if you don't do your job." Ninnies, they actually carded him before reattaching heart monitor gizmos to cart him off, siren pulsing, lights strobing.

I went to the back porch. My brother pretended he'd slept through the whole extravaganza. I thought of the fountain pen, the locked diary, the smashed van, and everything else. I don't need this, I said to myself, I'm getting out of here. I fished the rental car keys out of my purse.

He opened his eyes. "Where you going?" Like he'd been the host with the most and couldn't feature why I'd leave his terrific party.

"Your boyfriend had a stroke or something," I said. "Paramedics took him away."

"Finally! I threw out his pills a week ago," he said, and then as if by explanation, "what kind of co-dependent sicko sticks around to take care of a goner like me?"

He was dead serious. I couldn't leave now. "You are pure evil." I sat down.

"Thenk yoo," he leered, baring canines. "Thenk yoo veddy much." He shifted onto his side, diapers shooshing across the vinyl chaise cover. He closed his eyes again.

I thought of the snake, the poison oak, the broken locket. Smoke drifted to us from a neighbour's barbecue. People think they know what they'd save from a fire. They think they'd save important documents, mementos, family photos. No, what you take away from flames swarming curtains and wallpaper is how hair smells, burning. Wails, sirens filling the distance.

I considered hellfire, the nature of forgiveness and its practical applications before deciding against it as a viable option in this case.

My brother roused. "You're still here," he said.

"Look who's talking."

He turned onto his back. "I called you because there's something I want to tell you before I buy the farm," he said. "You'll be happy to hear it."

History made me wary. "I doubt it."

"I'm not your brother," he said. "We're not even related."

I thought of the rotten peaches, the lawyer's black Caddie glinting in the sun as it idled at the stop sign. Of my brother's ripe flesh, now turning to soft fermentation. That cold hard pit at his core was the only thing anchoring him. My brother, the stone fruit.

I lip-farted a *pffffft*. "That's it? That's your news flash? I'd be relieved, if it were actually true."

He was insulted. "I was old enough to remember my father bringing you home," he sputtered. "One of his teenage patients got knocked up and he wanted to help. He didn't believe in abortion. Plus, it was illegal then."

I knew I had him. "You think he made a fortune from sore throats and penicillin? Wrong, Sherlock. Dad made a fortune from his medical practice *because* abortion was illegal." Our father was the best abortionist in town. All the college girls came to him. Once it was legalized, the price dropped into the basement, and he was out of business. "He brought me home because one of his teenage patients was knocked up," I said, "and he was the one who knocked her up. So he was my father, too. Although it would be a comfort to know that you and I weren't drowning in the same gene pool."

People don't want the truth. They would rather have interesting facts: If this were Jupiter, we'd be eighty times heavier; Chester Greenwood patented ear muffs on March 13, 1887; everyone alive has taken in Caesar's last breath, because there are only so many molecules of air on earth for us all to inhale. You see? You can't tell the difference between truth and the facts I made up. What I said about my father was actual fact, but also the truth.

Show me a few people who can't tell the difference between truth and the facts—religious nut-cases, from ranting right-wing Armageddonists, to orange-robed woo-woos spouting, *If you are attached to anything, you will suffer*—and I'll show you people who are happy only when they're miserable.

My therapist, on the other hand, repeats the mantra that my lack of attachment causes my suffering. Who asked you anyway, I told him, did I mention the word *therapist* is a compilation of *the* and *rapist*? You see what I mean, he said, what lengths you'll go, to push help away? Good thing I don't need any help then, I told him, I just pay you every week so you can learn how the other half lives.

My brother pretended to doze, perhaps planning the next plot twist. I thought of the dog shit and the trash can fire and the secret tape recording.

But he said nothing more, even when I left. What is the purpose of pain—I slit open this vein of thought while window-shopping in the house—isn't it all illusory?

I am not the kind of person who steals for fun. Injuries I sustained years ago caused pains that endure in my back, sometimes also the heart. And pain is how you know you're alive, I decided. Although one might question the practical benefit of knowing you're alive, if living is defined by the awareness of pain.

There it was, big as life: palliation. His morphine sulfate pills, right on the kitchen counter.

You see how it was a win-win? He had to feel pain, in order to know he was still alive. I, being clearly alive, a condition whose defining characteristic is suffering, needed relief. Was I not entitled? *Thank you for your generous albeit passive hospitality, my so-called brother,* I thought, as I emptied his morphine into the Vicodin bottle I carry in my purse.

I am not cruel. I left him the tiny white pills I'd found at the airport in a fanny pack, briefly untended. Sadly, these had no effect on me, but if sharing my bounty can help another, I am happy to do it.

I knew I'd done the right thing—Vicodin plus morphine, that castanet rattle of pills against plastic, drowned out the sound of my heart.

Pat Cason is a psychiatrist living and working in rural northeast Oregon.

All Out of Funny in Crystal Lake, California

Stephan Clark

DEAR ABBY:

First off, let me say I've never done this before, so if you find yourself needing to edit for length or content, you just go right ahead. From what I've read of you this last year, you sound like a real reasonable woman. Smart too.

Now the reason I'm writing is Feeling Helpless in El Segundo, California. That woman sure has had it rough, Abby. First she loses her son Jesus in a drive-by (which is reason enough not to go naming your boy after the Lord), and then her husband's arthritis acts up and keeps him out of that mariachi band. I'll tell you, when I heard that, I just had to do something, and so now I'm writing this. It's not much, I know, but it's all I can offer, and at least maybe it'll show that woman she's not alone.

This evening I'd like to start, I came home to find Junior plopped down and drooling on the living room floor with one side of his diaper peeled away. Smelled something awful, Abby, he did. But I'd just punched the clock—my dogs were barking, I'm saying—so I walked right on over to the La-Z-Boy and turned on the tube. That puts me in a bad light, I know. No man should walk by his son, giving him little more than a quick rub on the head and a sad shake of his own. But you gotta understand. I thought Rosie'd be coming home soon. I thought maybe she'd just snuck out for a pack of her GPCs or a pint of that Canadian whisky she loves. So yeah, you could say I was ignoring my boy, which I hear's all but a prison crime these days, but you could just as easily say I was counting to ten. And I heard that on Oprah the other day. Says you gotta count that high to keep from getting angry. It works too. Round about eight I usually stop seeing red.

I was angry, though. Junior was born funny, you see. And I know that's not the way to put it, but if a doctor had ever told me any different, I'd be telling you the same now. We had that damn state insurance, you understand, and so far as I can figure it, it don't pay for much more'n the slap on the ass. My son's problems were plain to see, I thought. He came out looking all wrong. And I'm not saying I'm Tom Selleck, because I'm not. I got a face like one of them stones on that island, and my hair's all thick and red, which I guess works for some people. But Junior came out looking like he was from another planet, not just the back of the line. Grab the picture I sent you. You'll see. He's got so little chin he's gonna need help changing a pillowcase when he's older. And those ears? I find myself trying to pull'em up damn near every day, to say nothing of his nose. Will you look at it, Abigail? It's like a razor blade with a cherry stuck on one end.

And yet still not one doctor said a thing. He was delivered, they gave him the slap, and then out the door he went. State insurance, you know. It didn't get no better either. When we got him home, Junior wouldn't suck on Rosie or the plastic nipple. To get him to eat, Rosie had to pour that formula right on down his throat. I couldn't stand to watch. He'd get to bawling so bad I'd turn the volume up on the TV till whoever was talking there sounded like they wanted us to evacuate. Finally when he did take to the bottle, half the formula came right out his nose. I guess if he did it, he did it poorly or late. Sitting, crawling, walking, talking—everything. His first words weren't no different. They were ma-ma, Abby. But they were to me, the man of the house. He called his mother ball. So yeah, excuse me when I say it, but he was born funny. And whenever Rosie started bending down in front of him, saying, "C'mon, say ball, say ball," I guess we turned a little funny too.

Those doctors, though, they really burned my butt. They took all these tests, telling us Junior was slow, and had asthma, and was born with two holes in his heart, and had a weakened immune system, and a cleft palate, and was obsessive-compulsive, and then they said Rosie must be neglecting him, that she must be watching *Jeopardy* instead of dangling something bright and shiny in front of his face. Fuck them, Abby. Excuse me and edit that out, but fuck them. That's just me expressing myself, and that's another Oprah says.

Anyways, looking back I can see how Rosie maybe got to blaming herself. Because I'll admit it, I felt half-happy to hear a professional man say it wasn't my fault. I'm ashamed of that now, but it's true. Half-happy I wasn't the one to blame. Which brings me back to that day when Junior was just a-sitting there with his diaper half-peeled away. When Rosie still hadn't shown an hour later, I all but crawled inside the TV. The Giants were playing the Dodgers that day, and those boys in blue just had me tickled pink. Hideo Nomo, Raul Mondesi, Wilton Guerrero, and Chan Ho Park—it was like they were the United Nations, not some team from Los Angeles. Damn near only white guy they had was Mike Piazza, and he's Italian. But then it was the final out and Rosie was still gone and the room got soft and dark. I turned off the TV and just sat there. I can't stand that new guy who does the *Family Feud*.

It was a rough night. A rough couple of nights and weeks, I should say. I hit the bottle, for one. And I know that's not what you're supposed to do, but it's still what I did. I'd go on down to the Driftwood and drink my Oly and roll dice until I sometimes couldn't even pay the babysitter. Not that she was worth a damn anyway. That girl was a doper, Abby, just sixteen and with all the smarts of a dried-up houseplant. One evening I came home to find her having her way with my glue-gun. Damn near everything I owned was stuck to my living room wall, Abby. Bills, Pop Tarts and Fiddle-Faddle, my Elvis Presley bourbon bottle, and even the red bandanna I caught when Willie Nelson came through town. It was a sight, and so right then and there I told her off. I said, "Girl." And I looked at her too. I said, "Girl. I won't have no speed-freak watching my son. Now get. You hear me? Get!"

I didn't have to point long before she was out the door, and then I was left looking down at my boy. Junior's head was tilted back a-ways, and you could hear him kind of gurgling the spit that had collected in the back of his throat. He was bouncing his hands together too, which is something he does every now and then but never too well. Right as you think his hands are gonna meet, he pulls 'em back and starts all over again. It's funny, like he's playing patty-cakes but doesn't know how. So that night I told him, "Boy, that ain't how it's done." And I got on down on my knees. I did, Abigail. I got on down on my knees and showed him how to clap, pressing his hands together until they met. "See?" I said. "You feel that?" And he just grinned and gurgled and went right on back to clapping the empty air. "Shit," I said. And I wish I'd said something else now that I'm telling you, but that's what I did right there in front of him. I just looked at my boy clapping like he does, and I said to myself, "Shit," as if it were the most beautiful thing in the world.

Things picked up after that, and then one afternoon down at the Snatch 'n' Save a kind of miracle happened. I can't remember what I bought, but while this pretty young clerk was scanning me through, she asked if my boy had a condition. I moved Junior from one arm to the other and told her no, but she came right back and said he might have a genetic defect. "What makes you so smart?" I said, and she said, "Not saying I'm smart, just that he might have a defect." Junior kind of laughed then, as if he knew something was going on. I asked her, "Don't you think the doctors would've thought of that?" and she folded her arms and just looked at me as if I was the one born funny. "You'd be surprised," she said.

And I was too. The next day at the public library I got one of the women there to help me with the Internet. All it took was but a few minutes of searching and typing and then there it was, something called DiGeorge's syndrome. The ears, the chin, the nose—it was all the same, Abigail, and right then and there I knew that that's what my boy had. DiGeorge's syndrome. Put a name to it, you know. And that's something. A start at least.

That night I parked outside the Snatch 'n' Save waiting for the girl to get off work. I was afraid she was gonna think I was some kind of pervert, but when she came breezing through the glass doors and saw me, she came right on over and leaned down into the open window.

"It's DiGeorge's syndrome," I said, lifting the papers I'd printed out.

"That right?" she said.

I told her it was, and then I asked if she'd like to get a pizza. She cocked her head to one side and squinted as if trying to decide if this was sexual. She must've decided it wasn't, because she said, "You gonna let Junior sit on my lap?" and I told her, "You best ask him." We looked at him, then, sitting there on the front seat beside me, and he kind looked up and made his gurgling noise while clapping the empty air like he does. "I think he likes you," I said.

That girl was pretty smart, Abigail. She read what I'd brought her and told me Junior was missing a little chunk of his DNA. Said it was from the second-smallest of twenty-three pairs of human chromosomes, the one they call the twenty-two. Said the part of my boy that was missing moved on down to another chromosome, the number ten, none of which made much sense to me until she put it like this: "It's like when he was being made, someone attached his carburetor to the exhaust pipe." And let me tell you, my eyes just about jumped outta my head on that. I mean, a carburetor don't got no business being on an exhaust pipe, not even on a Chevrolet.

In the weeks that followed, the girl made some calls to the county and found out there was a way the state would pay her to take care of Junior. The money isn't much, but it's almost the same as what she pulled in at the Snatch 'n' Save, and she likes the work some. Most nights I get in late off the road and find her sleeping on the sofa with my boy in her arms. She's really something. Sweeter than a peach and prettier than a pear, my momma used to say. And no funny stuff goes on either, Abby. She's almost twenty years younger'n me, her whole life still a tray of wet paint. Wants to go off to the junior college, she says, and study nursing. So yeah, nothing funny. If I ever get to feeling something that won't go away, I just reach for a dirty magazine. I'm a changed man, I'm saying. Rosie'd be surprised.

But you really should see her. Some nights when she puts Junior away she tells him bedtime stories even though he can't understand. They ain't normal stories either, not the ones you and me grew up with at least. This one she favours is all about the Human Genome Project. She tells him it's the biggest thing since the A-bomb, and that all these smart fellas from all over the world are working non-stop to map out the millions of parts that go into our DNA. "It's a scientific revolution," she says, "and pretty soon they're gonna be able to twist and tinker and play around with our insides until all the funny's gone, maybe even before we're born."

Now, I don't know where you stand on that, Abby. I was raised Baptist myself. But something about it keeps me standing in the doorway listening. It gets to me every night. Come the end of her story, my boy brings his hands together and almost claps. And he's gonna do it one of these days too. That's what I'd like you to tell that lady in El Segundo. Tell her one day Junior's gonna clap, and when he does, it's really gonna be something.

 Sincerely,
 All Out of Funny in Crystal Lake, California

Stephan Clark has an essay in the forthcoming issue of Swink. It is part of a planned book about Ukraine, where he is currently living on a Fulbright Fellowship and researching the "mail-order bride" phenomenon.

911

Diane Foley

In my mind, schizophrenia is the worst illness anyone can have. If you have diabetes, you know you need a shot of insulin a day, but when your mind is ill, you are unable to perceive what's needed.

Guy's illness was getting worse. He was filthy. He wouldn't bathe. As soon as he entered a room, you could smell him. His breath stank. He was getting aggressive. Even the way he walked stated, "Don't touch me!" He was the proverbial orangutan.

For whatever reason, I was always his target. The one he loved the most.

I would phone the Mental Health Division for help, but because of the Mental Health Act, unless a mentally ill patient is a danger to himself or to another, he cannot be hospitalized against his will or forced to take medicine. So I had to wait helplessly until Guy became so deranged that he was capable of attacking me or somebody else.

No mother should be made to watch her son become an animal.

Now Guy had decided he didn't want to sleep in his own place anymore. Instead he insisted on crashing on our chesterfield every night.

Part of this was due to his paranoia. He thought he was being watched by the CIA. If a plane went overhead, he would rush to hide behind a bush, or if inside, behind a curtain. He felt safer in our house at night, but we had gone through two weeks of this and Larry's patience was wearing thin.

If only Guy would just go to sleep, who would care? But no . . . instead he would have the TV on until 3 a.m., and the worst of it was that his body odour, like rotting garbage, would come wafting into our bedroom.

Sometimes we would jolt awake to the sounds of banging pots and his laughter, as he cooked up leftovers. That loud, manic, incessant laughter.

To say it was wearing and disturbing doesn't quite conjure it up. It was the laughing of a madman, and we lay awake night after night nervous and afraid, waiting for something insane to happen—*insane* being the key word.

I kept asking him to go home. He lived three minutes away in a cabin that Larry had renovated. The cabin was as cute as button with a beautiful walk-in glassed shower, unused. It boasted the usual bachelor setup with a kitchen, living space, and bedroom all in one room.

Perfect for Guy.

But Larry was spitting nails now. Angry because Guy had turned everything on its side. His bed was tilted with bricks underneath; all the pictures on the walls were askew. When you walked in, the sight stopped you dead in your tracks. Van Gogh came to mind! Maybe I should buy him an oil painting kit.

Davey wanted to take pictures of the room to enter in a photo competition.

"It's a work of art, in a weird way," he said. "I kinda like it. It looks so different. It's artsy-fartsy, Diane," his laughter making him choke on his cigarette, thinking he was cute at stealing one of my favourite expressions.

But Larry was not so forgiving, seeing the fridge had been turned on its side and was now ruined.

"How the hell did he get it over like that? he puzzled, hands on hips, looking at the fridge sideways on bricks. "Your son must be as strong as an ox!"

Now here was Guy again, belligerent, yelling at me in our living room. "I don't want the pope visiting here—do you understand?"

"Guy, the pope's visiting Vancouver. He's not coming over to the Island, I swear to you."

"You're lying!" Spittle on his lips, his eyes wild. "Religion is evil. The pope is evil—don't you get it?" He slammed his fist on the coffee table, making us all jump like acrobats.

Larry stood up. "OK, Guy—I want you to go home now. Just go home and calm down."

With one quick movement, Guy jumped over the coffee table and had Larry up against the wall, his hand on his throat. "Don't you talk to me like that, you asshole. This is my mother's house. I'm not going anyway."

He pushed away from Larry and smashed his fist into the wall, leaving a hole. "I don't wanting the fucking pope here, and that is that." His face was purple.

I stood trembling by the door. Larry was white as a sheet. I made up my mind and tiptoed down the hall and called 911.

"My son has schizophrenia. He's not on meds, and he's getting violent—please hurry."

The police arrived in fifteen minutes. We could have all been dead.

They have a special police car for psychiatric incidents called Car 87. I had nicknamed it the Swat Team. Special police crews trained to handle psychotic behaviour were teamed up with a mental health nurse. Tragedy can still happen, and eight mentally ill people have been shot and killed by police in past years in BC.

Larry and I were questioned. Guy always keeps silent in front of the police, an internal radar system warning him to keep quiet.

The police finally took Guy away to hospital. They have to make sure that he is a danger to someone or himself, or the hospital won't accept him.

We all sat around, shaken and unhappy. I could barely look at Larry. He had always been so patient with Guy. I hoped he understood that Guy was really fond of him. Difficult to explain that to a man who has just been attacked.

Ken and Mr. D were patting Larry on the back. "Come on, Big Man, let's take you over to the Pat for a beer."

Larry still looked so white and shaken. I went over to him.

"Thanks for not hitting him back." I kissed him on his forehead. Though it would have been an involuntary reaction, Larry with his size and strength could have dropped Guy with one punch.

"Go on—have a beer with the boys. I'm ready for bed anyway. I've had enough of today."

I lay in bed in a half twilight sleep. I had woken up thinking that I'd heard the front door open. Were the guys back from the pub already? I peered through the dim light.

A figure standing at the end of the bed, watching me intently, motionlessly. I felt the hairs stiffen on the back of my head.

"You bitch," he said. "I'm going to off you—you bitch! You shouldn't have taken his side."

I froze in the dark. It was Guy. Why was he here?

"What happened at the hospital, Guy? Why are you here?" I kept my voice normal. I didn't want to trigger anything.

"They said I was OK. I am OK, you bitch!" he screamed the words so loudly, so viciously that my body jackknifed, lifting me off the bed. There was a glint of something in his hand.

Please dear God, let the boys come home soon, fast. Larry hurry! Then Guy walked out of the room saying, "I'm going to take a bath."

He wasn't allowed to do that in this house. Maybe, I thought, on some subconscious level he knew his lack of hygiene was tied in to proving the existence of his illness.

Only when I heard the water stop running and heard faint splashing in the tub did I tiptoe out of the bedroom to the hall. I strained in the dark to see the telephone dial and dialled 911. It seemed forever before someone answered. I went to talk and found my voice had left me. When I am on emotional overload that can happen. My throat was frozen.

"Help," I tried.

Surely they could pick my address on their computer. Didn't an incoming call pull up an address?

"Please speak up."

"Attack," I said. "Hurry," straining to hear if sounds of water in the bathroom were still splashing.

"Your address?"

Dear God, didn't they have computers in Nanaimo!

"55 Haliburton. Hurry, please." My voice was the tiniest croak.

Last time the police had taken fifteen minutes to arrive. Oh God! I was so afraid. Maybe they wouldn't get here in time. I hung up and called the Pat and asked the girl who answered to get a message to Larry or Ken, Ken being the best known there because of his singing on talent nights. My voice was still whispery but the waitress seemed to understand.

"I've got it. An emergency, tell them to get home fast."

I could see through the kitchen that the bathroom door was ajar.

"Mum—what are you doing?" I froze. Act normal—don't show any fear. Guy was out of the bath with a towel wrapped around him, dripping water on the kitchen floor, a carving knife held casually by his side.

"Get back to bed, you stupid bitch." He was snarling, baring his teeth.

I heard the front door open, footsteps running down the hall, Larry's arms coming out of nowhere grabbing me, the police coming in right after him, their bulk and their uniforms filling the kitchen.

They took Guy away, handcuffed, with just a towel around him. He was saying as they pushed him in the police car, "I just didn't want the pope to come here! What's all this fuss about?"

The phone was ringing. It was Guy's mental heath nurse, Karen. She explained why the hospital had not admitted him: "He holds it altogether so well at the hospital. He told them that he'd argued with Larry and it was just a family dispute. The admitting doctor bought into it. They are so strict about admitting someone unless they're violent, and Guy talked to them softly like a choirboy. He'd had time to calm down while he was waiting in Emergency, and well... he pulled it off, Diane. It's so frustrating. At least now they will admit him."

"The whole system stinks—he needs help, and they worry whether he is really dangerous? I wonder what their definition of dangerous is."

One day, I thought recalling the figure at the bottom of my bed, the police are going to be too late, and schizophrenia disguised as my son is going to kill me.

Diane Foley, a single mother of four children, lives on the Sunshine Coast of BC. Her eldest son was hit with schizophrenia at the age of seventeen. She is interested in world politics and loves to travel.

Stoma

Kathie Giorgio

Erin couldn't believe that just two months ago she wanted to climb on him one last time, soothe him, remove and keep a part of him with her in case he didn't come back as he went into a surgery neither of them expected. She smiled at him as he was rolled away, told him she'd see him later, tried to convince herself even as she convinced him. But as soon as his cart turned the corner, she leaned against the beige hospital wall and cried. A diverticulitis rupture was something she never considered when her thoughts turned dark on the evenings he was late. She pictured the various ways she could lose him. A heart attack, certainly, a stroke, a car crash, cancer, even suicide. But it was his colon, inflamed and angry, that simply chose to blow apart, filling his entire abdomen with infection. While the doctor was cheerful and upbeat with Jeffrey, he was matter-of-fact with Erin. "This is dangerous," he said. "He might not pull through." And Erin heard those words and their weight pulled at her shoulders, twisted her ankles. She stumbled as she walked down the hall and the doctor reached out to steady her. She wanted him to steady Jeffrey. "I just thought you should be prepared," the doctor said.

As if the slim ten minutes she had with Jeffrey before he was taken away would ever be enough to prepare. He was only forty, they'd been married only five years, she was barely prepared for their life, let alone his death.

Yet he made it through. There were eight weeks of recovery, of catheters and drains and IVs and oxygen and three different prescriptions for antibiotics, two for painkillers, and two more anti-nausea drugs. The top of their refrigerator went from a dust-filled catch-all to a pharmacy. And now his sweetly rounded stomach was S-scarred and there was a colostomy bag right where she used to rest her head.

The end of his colon stuck out through the upper left side of his abdomen, an odd mud-coloured extra belly button. The nurse told them it was called a stoma. Jeffrey called it Mick because he said it looked like Mick Jagger's lips. Erin hated the Stones and she hated even more the thought of Mick vomiting like a geyser, a volcano, into the special bag stuck to her husband's skin with paste and tape and a special elastic band he called his bra. It reminded her of the old menstruation belts she wore before pads stuck to her panties with adhesive strips. She remembered how uncomfortable it was and now Jeffrey was uncomfortable too.

Mick was uncontrollable. She and Jeffrey sat down to supper and suddenly he'd get a strange look on his face and he'd pat his shirt. "What's wrong?" Erin said every time, even though she knew the answer, but since his illness, she always had to know if he was okay. "Mick is singing," he answered and Erin would swallow, then clear her plate from the table. It was hardly dinner music.

They never even used the toilet in front of each other. They never even left the bathroom door open. It was something they agreed upon before their marriage. Erin was married before, for seventeen years, and she told Jeffrey that she felt part of that failure was too much familiarity. "He came in and used the toilet while I was brushing my teeth, showering, getting ready for work. He talked to me above his own noise. And sometimes when it was me on the pot, he'd stand by the sink and wait for me to finish. 'Don't flush,' he always said, 'let's save on the water bill.'" Jeffrey agreed that there were some things that should be kept private.

But now there was Mick, and Mick had no sense of privacy. He was always there, a singer whose toxic stage was her husband's stomach. Jeffrey never left the bag off for long because Mick's concerts were unscheduled and unpredictable.

And now, two months later, Jeffrey, with Mick at his side, was hinting toward the resumption of their intimate life. Passing by, he touched her, smoothed her shoulder, patted her bottom, kissed her neck. When she brushed her hair in front of the dresser mirror, her arms raised to the back of her head, he slid behind her, embraced her breasts, pressed himself against her and she heard the crinkle of plastic. At night, his caresses became less subtle and she carefully tucked his hand away, claiming fatigue, a headache, an early morning.

His touches were a question that she knew she had to answer soon.

In the hospital, the nurse showed them how to clean the stoma, saying it had no feeling. And Mick certainly didn't, though Erin constantly reminded herself that her husband did. The five years of their marriage seemed amazingly short, the rest of their lives together stretched interminably long as Mick followed them everywhere, out to dinner, to the movies, to bed at night. They didn't even have children, yet they were now a threesome. Erin, Jeffrey, and Mick. Wife, husband, and stoma.

She and Jeffrey talked about sex once, soon after he came home from the hospital. At the time, she didn't think it would be a problem, she was so happy to have him, so happy to see him relaxed in his chair in the living room, seated at her right in the kitchen, lying to her left in the bed. All of those spaces could have been vacant, and she wanted only to hug him, to prove to herself that he was still there, still whole, still warm and breathing steadily. In the hospital room, before and after the surgery, she wanted him, and if she could have, she would have raised the stiff white sheets to his waist and straddled him, took him into herself so she could feel his sameness, feel that he was still altogether and in one piece. But he was in such pain then, and she contented herself with kissing him as gently as possible. Through his pain, he still smiled, and in his smile and the softness of his voice as he called her name, she recognized everything she could have lost. On that first night home from the hospital, she said, "I don't know if I can handle feeling the bag against me," and he promised to wear a shirt, a cloth barrier between her and Mick. It seemed a small thing, a simple solution, and she was elated.

But it was a barrier to Jeffrey as well. He wore a shirt to bed every night and she never felt the warmth of his chest against her bare back or pressed against her breasts. There was always cloth. And there was always Mick. At any time, a look could cross Jeffrey's face and he touched his shirt and Erin wished she could shut a door.

ERIN STOOD in front of her dresser, looking down at the open drawer. It was filled with the never-worn nightgowns she received at a wedding shower. She always slept naked with Jeffrey and now she wondered if that should change. Maybe her nakedness was sending the wrong message, making it even harder on Jeffrey than it should be. Maybe it made her too accessible. She pulled out a nightgown, examined its lacy pink sheerness, but then put it back. It was just more cloth. Jeffrey would notice if she wore it. And then he would ask and she didn't want to answer.

She heard Jeffrey coming up the stairs, so she quickly slid into bed, pulling the sheet and blanket up to her neck. Jeffrey moved into his accustomed spot behind her, nuzzled her neck, then began to touch her breasts. He was naked from the waist down and she felt him harden against her hips. Gently, she tucked his hands at her waist and tried to put a smile in her voice. "Time to go to sleep, hon," she said. That used to be enough.

But now he said, "Erin, I want you." His hands twitched and slid down her thighs. She quickly crossed her legs.

"It's late," she said.

He froze, then pushed away. His sigh filled the room with an air so black, Erin closed her eyes to hide from it. Holding very still, she hoped that would be the last of it, that he would inhale and the light would return and they'd say their usual goodnights. But then he said, "Is this the way it's going to be?"

She rolled onto her back and opened her eyes. She waited for her vision to adjust, until she could see the white glow of their ceiling, surreal in the dark. "I don't know," she said.

"It's still me, Erin," he said.

She nodded. "I know. But you're not alone. There's him too."

"Him?"

"Mick." She tried not to cry, she didn't want to add tears to this mess. It was Jeffrey that nearly died, she reminded herself, Jeffrey that went through the pain and Jeffrey that would live with Mick twenty-four hours a day for the rest of his life. It wasn't her problem, Mick wasn't really her problem. Think of Jeffrey. "It's just . . ." She couldn't think of a way to end the sentence. "I don't know."

His voice was quiet. "I don't like him either. He doesn't make me feel the most attractive, you know."

She thought of Jeffrey fully dressed, khakis, polo shirt, his neat white sneakers he actually polished. No sign of Mick anywhere. She bought him shirts a size larger so that there was no cling, just soft folds that he tucked beneath his belt so the bag's corners and creases were hidden. "You are attractive. You know that. I see you and I just want to touch you. You know I love touching you. But then . . ."

There was a rustle and a crinkle and she knew he was patting Mick. "Then you see him."

"Yes." She sat up suddenly. "I want you to touch me, not him. I want to be with you, not him. But no matter what we do, he'll be there, touching me somewhere. Me on top, you on top, sideways, you behind me, he's still there and he'll be against me. And what if he goes off, Jeffrey? What if he sings? What will be against me then?"

His voice went flat. "The same thing that's against me until I go the bathroom and empty him."

She felt chilled. And she felt small, like she just folded into herself, in half and in half and in half again until she was just one little scrap in the bed. So she tried, she kissed Jeffrey, pressed herself against his side, felt his fingers flutter over her nipples, then slide down her stomach. She opened her legs, tried to feel desire, tried to picture Jeffrey over her, his face strained and ecstatic, but all she could see was Mick, his mouth open and gagging, and she imagined the plastic cold against her skin turning suddenly warm. Abruptly, she broke away. "Jeffrey, I can't." She rolled onto her side, drew her knees up, crossed both arms over her breasts. "I just can't."

Jeffrey groaned, but moved away. In the dark, she held her breath and tried not to listen as Jeffrey masturbated next to her, finally coming with a sound like a puncture.

SHE WOKE to a feeling of warmth, of wetness, and her own soft and intimate sounds. It was still dark, she was on her back, and Jeffrey's fingers were sliding over her, inside of her, in all the ways that she liked. She jerked to alertness but he slung one leg over hers and whispered, "Don't move. Just enjoy." And because her body was already well ahead of her mind, already on edge and teetering, she arched her back and opened her legs further. He kept a steady rhythm, moving no faster, no slower, in the maddening way he knew she liked, and he began to whisper into her neck, just below her ear, his breath warming her and bringing every hair up and rigid. "God, I want you, Erin, I love you, I want to be inside you, I want to feel you come, Erin, I want to feel you come around me, I want to feel the throb that is all mine, all mine, that is all because of me..."

Her build was slow and delicious and she wondered if he would stop, the way he always did, just before she peaked, if he would stop and tease her with a long kiss to keep her from begging him out loud to enter her. And she wondered what she would say, if he tore his lips away, if she would beg, if she would want him there.

His hand paused and there was his kiss and she caught her breath, waited for her voice, but nothing came out but a moan, a sad sound, and then his hand was back, bearing down and she came hard, blindingly hard, all sensation and colour and wonder.

But when it was over, when her body relaxed, she realized her legs didn't want to close, that her arms were reaching out, and without a voice, she urged him up and onto her. He didn't say anything either, but as she locked her legs around his hips and drew him in, she saw him smile and she recognized that smile, recognized all that she could have lost but didn't, it was all still here, he was still here, and oh God, she still loved him. He kept his eyes open, watching her, and she smiled back, and then she ran her hands around his waist, found the hem of the shirt, and began pulling it upwards.

"Erin?" He paused in his rhythm and she heaved upward, demanding more. She grabbed him in a kiss, only releasing him long enough to yank the shirt over his head. And then she held his bare shoulders, pulling him down until his full weight was on her.

Mick was there. He pressed against her and she could feel he was flat. For a moment, all sensation telescoped onto him, onto the three by six inch slice of plastic that was cold and sharp and dead. But then she arched her back, squeezed her legs, pressed her breasts into his chest and rubbed her cheek against his and she felt Jeffrey everywhere. He was there, on every other surface, every other inch, and he was warm and moist and smooth rhythm and he was inside, filling her. She moved with him and when he came, it was with a sound that was at once raucous and joyful and wonderfully, fully alive.

They clung together in the aftermath until their bodies cooled. When

Jeffrey tried to roll away, Mick stuck to Erin, his plastic cemented by her sweat. Mick's brown unfeeling lips pressed against the side of the bag, and as Jeffrey carefully peeled him away, there was the pop of broken suction.

"Oh, yuk," Erin said quickly, involuntarily, and then she slapped both hands over her mouth. But Mick was gone, back to his own side of the bed, and Jeffrey took her hands, squeezed them, kissed her knuckles.

"Only one yuk," he said. "I can live with that."

And he could. Erin smiled at him and knew she could too.

Kathie Giorgio's stories have appeared in many national and international literary magazines. She is the director of AllWriters' Workplace & Workshop (www.allwriters.org) and the editor of Quality Women's Fiction *magazine. She is a happy overachiever.*

Unpacking My Daughter's Library

Joan Givner

I am sitting on the floor, surrounded by books in piles and in boxes, which I am unpacking. It is every book-lover's dream—to inherit a library. Yet this is one legacy I never expected, never would have wished for, partly because at my age it is more appropriate to bequeath books than to inherit them.

Not that there is anything of great value on my bookshelves. I am an accumulator rather than a collector and my shelves have more in common with a garage sale than a library. The reference books have been rendered useless by Google; the textbooks are out of date; and the hardcovers hover between obsolescence and antiquarian value.

Nevertheless when I retired, I drew up a will making careful arrangements for the disposal of the books. If I died on an even day of the month, my elder daughter was to make the first selection: if on an odd day, the younger one. Then turn and turn about, they would divide up the whole collection. The plan was designed to prevent strife, though I knew it was more likely to end in a tug of war.

In the event, it proved unnecessary.

One July evening, nine years later, a doctor at the Queen Elizabeth II hospital in Halifax called to tell us that our elder daughter had died of a sudden allergic reaction. It is her library that I am now unpacking.

Soon after the phone call, I flew across the continent to give the eulogy at my daughter's memorial service. Afterwards, I went directly to the house in which she had lived for the past two years. Her bedroom was just as she had left it when she walked out for the last time—a desk heaped with papers, letters, manuscripts of stories she was working on, and an overflowing bookcase. Shelves crammed with her books were all over the house. As my younger daughter said in her tribute, "The way Emily lived says much about what she thought was important. She spent little time collecting anything other than books."

I yearned to possess those books, but even I, desperate for every relic of her life, realized that to strip the house of her books would be a cruel blow to the artist with whom she had made a home. Instead I sorted out all the manuscripts, papers, and letters, packing some to carry home in my luggage, others to send by mail. The books remained behind.

The loss of books became a source of grief that compounded the greater loss of my daughter. It also became a festering source of resentment. In one of my daughter's stories was a scene in which two lovers were separating:

> She was packing her books, soft covers in one box, the critical theory in another, the antiquarian first editions in a giant milk crate.
>
> Rick had moved up behind her. Quietly. But she could feel his presence.
>
> "Could you leave the books here?" he asked.
>
> "Why, Rick?"
>
> "I like the look of them on my shelf."

I read that passage as a description of the present situation. Jim was a visual artist, who loved art more than literature, treasured paintings more than books. He liked the look of them on his shelves! I doubted that he would ever read them, and I feared the books would be borrowed and not returned, carried outdoors and left in the rain, given away as gifts to friends. I felt that I had been robbed of something precious. Neither the sense of deprivation nor the resentment diminished over the next four years.

Then, another turn of fate! Another tragic death! Jim had started out as an idealistic painter, unconcerned that his huge colour field canvases were too large even for most art galleries. Eventually, he was driven by necessity to earn a living by painting sets for movie companies. It was an expedient course that not only compromised his art, but destroyed

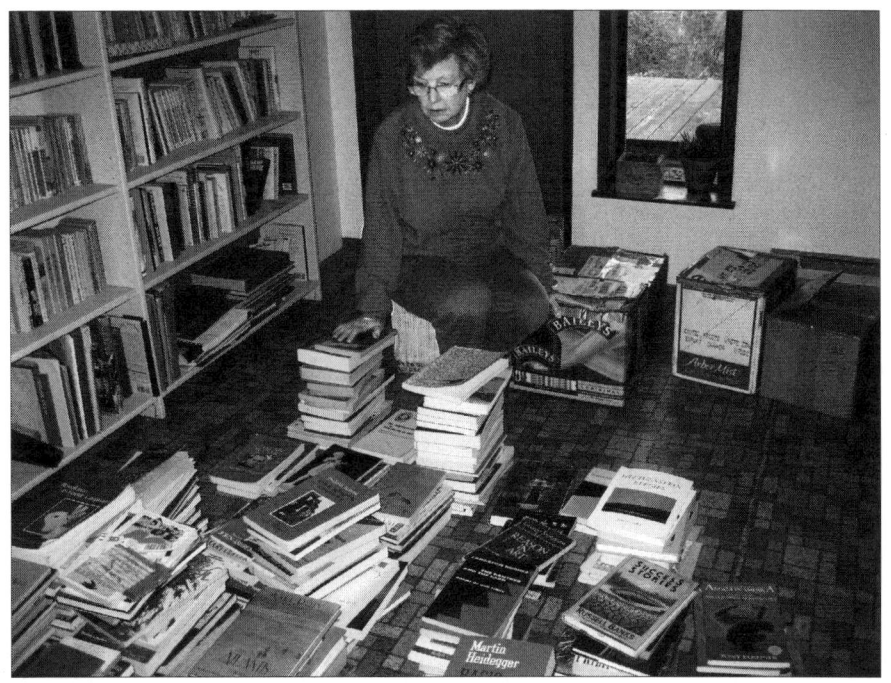

Joan Givner with the library of her daughter Emily

his health. He ruined his lungs by painting without a mask to protect against the toxic fumes and died of a pulmonary thrombosis.

And so my daughter's library was mine. It had been restored to me in a way I never would have wished; it was at the far end of the continent, and in a house soon to be dismantled. Then a small miracle! Out of the wings stepped someone I barely knew, had met only once—the wife of Jim's brother, herself a writer, a book-lover, a survivor of the Eastern European devastation. She offered to catalogue the books, pack them in boxes, and ship them to me. All this she did, sending them by a courier service to ensure their safety.

Her catalogue preceded the boxes and, I saw to my shame, that I had misjudged Jim. He had been a faithful custodian and had lovingly preserved Emily's library; not a single volume was lost. The list contained hundreds of books—high school and college textbooks, special editions of her favourite authors, and multiple copies of the same books by authors whose work she had needed when she travelled. She acquired them over and over again, wherever in the world she was, for Emily needed books, as others need food and clothing.

"A private library," Walter Benjamin tells us, "serves as a permanent and credible witness to the character of its collector." The library that was on its way to me contained Emily's biography. It traced the trajectory of her life—her college courses, teaching stints in Korea and Poland, brief literary infatuations, forays into philosophy and literary theory, and her enduring passion for poetry.

Above all, it was a writer's library. It spoke of what she had written and what she might have written, if she had lived awhile longer. A tattered paperback describing the lives of the Russian women pilots of the Second World War was the key to her story "Night Witches." The biography of Clement Greenberg together with the catalogue for a show of Marsden Hartley's paintings would help me understand "Fisherman's Last Supper." Book after book was able to yield new insights and allow me to engage once again in a dialogue with my daughter about the books we loved and the stories she wrote. I prepared for their arrival, as one might prepare for the arrival of a child, making a special space in the room where I am now sitting, clearing shelves and buying new ones.

And then, one final devastation!

Only a portion of the shipment arrived. In a panic, I made desperate calls to the parcel service. Days passed in nervous anticipation, but eventually the missing boxes arrived. The deliveryman, who was by this time taking a friendly interest in the situation, shook his head as he set them in the hallway. They felt odd and looked very strange—the sides had burst and been crudely taped back together. He stood looking down as I opened them. Instead of books, they contained heavy metal pieces that I was unable to identify. He called them "clamps."

I flew into action, confident that the lost books could still be traced. After all, if the clamps were in my house, the books must be in someone else's. The rightful owner of the clamps must be scratching his head at that very moment over a bunch of poetry books instead of the tools he needed to build whatever he was building. If not with him, the books must be in a shipping warehouse somewhere along the way.

I spoke constantly by phone to the representatives of the parcel service—young women called Randi, Rebecca, and Sherri. The verdict was horrifying: the parcel service had no responsibility for the books. I should contact the agent at the shipping office from which they had been sent. Besides, they were uninsured. I protested and pleaded. Surely the payment of hundreds of dollars constituted a guarantee of safe delivery. Not so: no insurance, no responsibility. Worse still, no interest at all in the recovery of the lost items.

That verdict made no sense to me. I assembled the necessary documentation: the tracking numbers on the boxes, shipping dates, lists of the missing books, and close-up photographs from all angles of the smashed boxes and the metal clamps. Nothing unlocked the colossal indifference of the parcel service and their refusal to trace the books. In voices resembling those of automated check-out clerks at the supermarket, Randi, Rebecca, and Sherri repeated the same lines. My long-suffering lawyer explained again and again about precedence, the legal system, and the futility of suing.

For weeks the boxes of clamps stood in the hall by the front door, the parcel service showing as little interest in picking them up as it had in finding my books. Presumably, their unfortunate owner, like me, had omitted to insure them.

As time wore on, those smashed boxes of clamps took on a monumental significance. They became the terrible emblem of everything I had suffered in the last five years, and of all those who inflicted so much pain—the vendor who sold the sandwich containing the deadly allergen (Emily always asked about ingredients), the 911 operator who dispatched an ambulance too late, the paramedics who arrived unprepared to save Emily's life, the coroner's receptionist who promised the autopsy report week after week but failed to send it until I hired a lawyer. All these griefs were revived and suffered again in a great landslide of remembered griefs.

The books never appeared.

I told myself they could not have been shredded, recycled, and destroyed completely. "They must be somewhere," became my mantra. They must be in a repository of lost property, dumped in a heap, dispatched to the Salvation Army. At last, I dreamed that they were salvaged in one's or two's; that they found good homes with readers who loved them, and marvelled at the treasures to be found in Thrift stores.

So many precious books down the ages have by some evil chance been thrown away, burned by zealots, whole libraries buried deep in the ocean or under layers of volcanic ash—the Dead Sea Scrolls, the poems of Sappho, the libraries of Alexandria and Herculaneum. Of seven centuries of poetry written by the Anglo-Saxons, little remains, save a few prayers, one great epic, some haunting lyrics, and a beautiful dream vision.

When I was twenty-one and a student of literature, I made the pilgrimage from Milan to an out-of-the-way town in northern Italy. There a trusting priest placed in my hands one of only four surviving Old English manuscripts—the Vercelli Book. All afternoon in the cool interior of the cathedral, I read "The Dream of the Rood." It was written, not in the Latin of the learned clerics, but in the vernacular, the language of my ancestors. I deciphered the ancient script, smiling at the droll little creatures doodled in the margins by a playful scribe, and I thrilled to that simple climactic line: "Crist waes on rode."

I wondered at the strange chance by which it came to be there, and the even greater miracle of its being there still. No one knows how it got there in the first place. Did some English nobleman, making a pilgrimage to Rome, lose it? Did he leave it there and plan to retrieve it later? Was it stolen from him? It was a book from a foreign country in an incomprehensible language. Soon its method of production was rendered obsolete by the invention of the printing press. Did it then become a curiosity? Was it valued, or just overlooked? There were so many chances for its destruction over ten centuries of plague and strife and two world wars. Yet there it was. And there it is.

Fifty years later, as I sit here among the remnants of my daughter's library, I remember that day. I hold in my hands Emily's high school copy of Tennyson's *Idylls of the King*. It is as precious and amazing to me now as the Vercelli Book was then. Opening it at the story of Lancelot and Elaine, I learn from the marginal notes that "black tarn" means "a glaciated lake," and that Lancelot values honesty. In my mind's eye I see her so clearly, fifteen years old, sitting in a classroom, her head bent over the book, then suddenly laughing at the neighbour who has leaned over to scribble in pencil on the page, "Hi Emily, you twit."

From a copy of *The Beautiful Mrs. Seidenman* by Andrzej Szczypiorski fall two photographs and a note from a friend:

Dear, dear M!
I'm sorry I'm sending this so late.
I loved the novel but this is some strange translation.
Hugs,
Kinga

I write Kinga and she tells me about the photographs. They were taken in spring at the Metropolitan restaurant, just off the main square in Cracow. Her son, Kajetan, was eating his first ice cream of the year. Emily was drinking her usual strong coffee. At the next table, Czeslaw Milosz was eating a club sandwich.

Thus every book in its own way yields up its secrets.

It seems that some small fragments always survive devastation to console us in our sorrow. They provide permanent and credible witness to times past and lives lost. They are what we find again when the fighting stops, the wars are over, the destruction ends, and the tides of ignorance and indifference recede.

They are our bulwarks against despair.

Joan Givner has written two biographies, an autobiography, several works of fiction, and the Ellen Fremedon series of YA novels. Her next one, A Girl Called Tennyson, *will appear in the fall.*

My Father's Polio

Patricia F. Goldblatt

On Labour Day Weekend 1948, when I was eighteen months old, my father came down with polio. He called a cousin who was a doctor because his own doctor was away, was upbraided for complaining, mowed the grass of his new house, and collapsed.

When I was in my teens, my mother parcelled out these details. She said that I stole a lozenge from his nightstand, one that he had recently discarded, too exhausted to even finish it. They had waited for signs of illness to appear in me.

She confided these morsels because I did not remember them. She showed me photos, and I gradually constructed meaning from them, imagining how the curly headed tot felt, beside the worn woman in a gingham dress and the seated man who appeared to have had the air punched out of him. Each seemed in a private world, separate, unable to relate. Each was as closed as a mussel shell. As an adolescent listening to these histories, I, too, was enclosed in an uncomfortable world, trying to piece together who I was, and what this tenuous relationship was with my strong-willed father.

As the stories of my developing life were disclosed, I recreated deeply hidden dread and pain that I thought an eighteen-month-old child might experience when her father disappeared for almost a year into Riverdale Isolation Hospital. I tried to relive a child's shock when ambulance sirens came and my father abruptly disappeared.

Could the adolescent-me understand her father's sardonic wit as he revealed that he could see public hangings from his hospital window? Was his rare confiding in me an attempt to bring father and daughter closer, or just a quiet recollection that somehow leaked out from darkling memories preferably forgotten?

As I approach sixty, I am attempting to locate phantom scenes from my past to explain my present. In bits, I try to recreate and better understand my relationship with my father through narratives that had been decanted to me like rare and bittersweet wines.

My mother often told me that she had visited my father in the hospital every single day for the nine months he was in that strange world populated by other polio victims. She had written letters every night, too, while working early morning hours as a bookkeeper.

En route to see my father, my mother would deposit me at my grandmother's, a detour from the hospital, and was admonished not to stop for coffee, but to come back as fast as she could to reclaim her child. It was a long ride from North Toronto by bus and streetcar, first to my grandmother's and then to Riverdale Hospital, but every day this frail but determined woman completed the cycle. Knowing how my father adored my mother, I surmised that her visits kept him going, the only time he might have smiled in the deadening routines that had become his life. From the moment he met her he had known that this was the girl he would marry.

When I was sixteen, I found correspondence from those black days in the bottom of a mahogany chest in their bedroom. His handwriting was shaky. He had learned to write with his opposite hand when polio destroyed his good one. He repeatedly commented on how terrible his writing was, but I did not respond, thinking that to agree would hurt and make him think I pitied him. He hated to be pitied. So I looked away. In my mind's eye, I want to look away from the image my mother shared of him rolling out of bed the first night he came home from hospital, muttering that he would have preferred to die.

There were so many things he had to relearn. Perhaps I thought I could come closer to this solitary man by emulating his cold, detached behaviour, keeping the hurt out of sight. Only as an adult could I realize that his impenetrable surface was armour to protect broken dreams. How could I calculate the impact of an illness on a man six feet tall, dark-eyed and curly headed with his life ahead of him, a person who at twenty-eight believed that his talents, good looks, and intelligence were enough to ensure a future of promise?

Once a drill bit deeply punctured his arm as he was making plates for the amplifiers he built and perfected for wealthy homes and university music labs. He got his jacket, said goodbye to my mother, and drove himself to the hospital, uncomplaining. I did not find this behaviour surprising.

Like a ghost who never leaves, polio had lingered in our home, returning when my father was in his sixties to remind him that any hard-won independence was to be sucked back, and ruined muscles would be further drained of energy, further atrophied. But in his sixties, he was brave, even valiant, swimming at Sunnybrook Hospital, even laughing a bit at the contraption that lifted him in and out of the pool. He loved to swim because he could stand and move by himself, unencumbered, in the pool. He was free of supports. It buoyed his spirits. He hated the ghost who had stolen his legs and weakened his once-powerful body.

A taciturn man, he covered any bare surface he could find with squiggles that resembled pieces of kinky hair. These knotted doodles represented innovations in circuitry in audio engineering. My father's pencil marks embellished the tops of cake boxes and the margins of magazines as he turned his thoughts into problem-solving diagrams. He would knit his brows and focus inward. Removed from the vagaries of daily living, he bent over his resistors, wires, tools, tubes, and circuit boards, unconcerned about appearances, time, or money.

He associated me with his least favourite sister. She talked about art in an elitist, affected jargon, pointing out to him, time and again, how uncouth, how uncultured he was. My mother confided other reasons for his contempt for her: that she would not help fund a trip to Georgia's Warm Springs where Franklin Delano Roosevelt had grown stronger. He never went.

My fledging art encouraged by his hated sister began to appear on phone books or random pads. He called my drawings "muckah-puckah." *His* drawings of electronic circuits were serious, productive. Being involved in the arts was an indictment, considered frivolous.

Yet one day he arrived home with a large and expensive art book that I had been wanting. The only place it was available was on Queen Street, a street so busy and inaccessible to a man on crutches—and long before handicapped parking—that I wondered how he had managed this quest. Stranger still, I could not fathom how he had carried it from the store, as he needed his hands to grip his crutches, while swinging his wasted legs.

He had practised swinging his legs from his hips, something else he had to relearn. The Sister Kenny method, my mother called it.

He merely handed the art book to me with a half smile, no words. So many years later, I can see him framed in the doorway. I managed to blurt out, "Oh Daddy, how did you know?" although I had spoken of nothing else since my art teacher had written down the name of the book. I accepted this gift as if my father were rich, able-bodied, knowledgeable in matters of art and in tune with the soul of a fourteen-year-old girl. I did thank him, but I did not kiss him.

Now I wish I had reached up to touch his stubbled cheek. I wondered if perhaps I had kissed him. Hoping

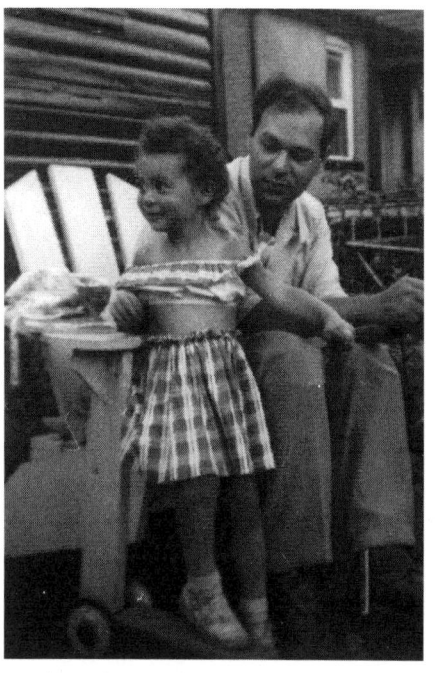

With my father, after his return from hospital

that my remembered surprise had erased this important detail, I asked my eighty-four-year-old mother. She confirmed the picture I had carved in my head: "No. You did not kiss him."

Did I feel I would embarrass him if I fussed, opening myself to another accusation of being too sensitive? Even today, I cannot revisit this memory without tears. My father often scolded me for being too sensitive, admonishing me, complaining that I cried too easily. When he sat beside me, teaching me chemistry or attempting to instruct me in how to drive a car, his voice was sarcastic, impatient with my slow learning, particularly in the sciences he adored.

Was I transfixed by his feat of acquiring the art book, tacitly knowing, even as an adolescent, the sheer enormity of the task? I wonder if he felt as if he had climbed Everest to bring me such a gift. I remember his quiet half smile. I, too, have always been quiet, loving words but preferring to write them and hear them in my head. I have his brown eyes, his beautiful smile. He smiled that day. I remember that.

Every day, he wore grey shirts and ties, grey pants. They set off his looks, Semitic, Spanish, Mediterranean, macho. He was solitary but not lonely, handsome even as he aged, totally absorbed by the work he loved. At his cluttered workbench, he was the picture of the watchmaker. Here he sat, free of the ghost that was never far.

As an adult, I can understand, at least intellectually, how a twenty-eight-year-old hunk of a guy would react with bitterness and scorn when the future had been altered forever. Not to be able to walk unaided ever again, literally brought to his knees, no, right to the ground, rendered helpless in his prime. In my imagination I want to curl up in his lap and say, "Daddy, I am here. I will help you." I apply the standards of today that parents are easy with hugs and kisses: more friends than strict progenitors.

He coped with his life; he made adjustments; he built things; he concocted machines; he worked at reshaping reality. He tinkered with cars and streamlined them, those keys to his independence. He polished them, keeping them pristine, unlike his cluttered workbench. Those cars were extensions of himself, his legs, to demonstrate that he could function as any man and support his family.

He drove every evening to install or repair his audio equipment and the televisions he sold. Sometimes he fell in the snow, his crutches sliding out from under him. He hated to be seen as vulnerable and prone, unable to hoist himself, yet refusing any help to pull himself erect again.

He had occasional helpers to carry his tools, but they were not serious workers. His expectations, his demands, and his intensity would have driven away most apprentices. I doubt he would have wanted to share the secrets of his trade, always impatient with those less talented than he.

He believed in his own superiority in his work, and he was right. Even as a little girl, I saw people coming and going to our store to consult with him, asking the most difficult questions that no one else could answer. He did not profit from this help he gave them. It was simply the pleasure of mentoring and expressing his knowledge. He savoured this intellectual exploration. He was the guru at Tele Sound, his shop, spending long hours in explanation, enjoying focused conversations. I stood in the hallway, transfixed by lively, passionate conversation, my father easily smiling, even laughing, approachable and friendly, a man I rarely knew.

I did not ask for stories, although I wanted to hear them. I wanted to listen to stories about me, my place in the scheme of things. Yet I feared the stories because I knew I could not hope for happy tales. I knew not to ask too many questions. There was a feeling, a look, words cut and measured carefully as if too many would cause things to spill out dangerously, causing pain, depression, and piercing silences.

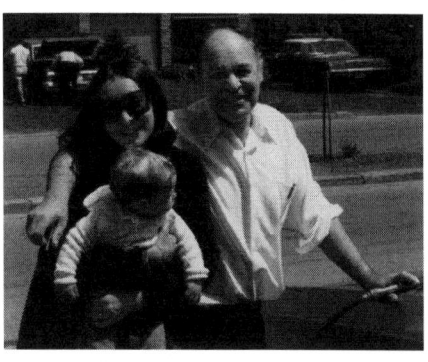

With my father and a grandchild

As I search for demonstrations of his outward affection for me, I cannot locate them in my memory. At sixty, I ask my mother, who also finds none. I know I must not try to understand him from a contemporary perspective, yet it is a quest to which I return when I seek solace and belonging. I continue to attempt to rearrange the fragments of stories in order to comprehend my father, and the polio that changed our lives.

The narratives are confusing and ambiguous, but I replay them in my head:

I had just turned two, on Christmas. I had not seen my father for four months since that Labour Day weekend, but because it was Christmas, I was permitted a visit. When we arrived, Big Nurse changed her mind and refused me a chance to be with my father. I was held up to a small window so he could see me. My mother told me that I cried at the window, cried on the long bus ride home, and cried myself to sleep from exhaustion.

An aunt told me there was a Christmas tree at the hospital, and to pass the time, she held me up to see the lights and decorations. I reached for a shiny red ornament and it shattered in my chubby palm. My aunt had to extract the slivers from my hand before my mother returned from seeing my father. She never told my mother of the incident. Indeed, in my mother's stories of my birthday visit, she never even mentioned my aunt.

The details of both tales seem realistic and appropriate: tree, ornament, window, Big Nurse. Both stories appear to be true. But I want to pry these morsels apart and discover more about myself. I want to know more details, but with each new crumb, I dive deeper into myself, experiencing deep ache.

In Grade 12, I wrote a story in my English class about a boy with polio, a boy who wore a St. Christopher's medal with which he squished the life out of insects. He perched on a hill, looking down on his school chums, watching them silently and mocking them. It was an outstanding story and my teacher told me to read it to the class, but I was shy and my voice shook so badly that when I took my seat, the teacher told the class that the reading had ruined the story

There was another bitter hospital narrative. It must have been my father who told it, as I can still feel how blackly he expressed his embarrassment to be held captive, almost naked, unable to move from an examination table, the topic of study as a former classmate, now an intern, accompanied the doctor at Riverdale Isolation Hospital. A fine specimen for polio investigation, they must have thought. I feel my father's pain, outrage, despair, a bug pinned to the wall. He had told me that as the nerves in his body were being destroyed by polio, he was able to project the unbearable pain onto a night table beside his hospital bed, detaching his mind from his body, deadening himself.

I have heard, but cannot know the extent of the medical miscalculations, humiliations, the disregard, the suffering endured by polio victims like my father. Yet these are stories I seek out to make my own, stories I cannot remember when or why I know.

My mother's strange words of consolation were to be thankful that he did not need an iron lung, because with his asthma, he would not have survived.

I was curious as a girl and rebellious as an adolescent, but as an adult I see threads that wind throughout my life. Always I wanted to know more about my father's illness, yet I needed to hold back, afraid to investigate because the knowledge I might find would only hurt.

As an annoying teenager, I wanted my father to be like everyone else's dad. I continued to plague him with the same question: "Why don't you wear madras shorts?" Finally exasperated, he spat out that his emaciated legs and ugly braces would be exposed. "Is that what you want?" he hurled at me, harder than any physical slap.

In spite of my mother's attempts to ensure that our life was normal, I can finally acknowledge that polio altered our family dramatically, making a hero of FDR, causing my mother to write to Russia in search of "the

Caucasian snowdrop" that might herald the cure to polio.

How late it is to stand outside of these stories and not be frightened by the tall man who towered above me, held erect by the two rubber-tipped sticks and braces halfway up his legs.

As I approach sixty, I can begin to forgive him for growing hardened, cynical, and distant, perhaps because he could not chase me into the garden, teach me to ride a bicycle, or swing me high into the air. My mother entreated my father, "Saul, tell her you love her." My father, weak from chemotherapy for his lymphoma, replied, "Of course I love you. You were my firstborn." I smiled weakly, then turned away.

My memories as a child are few and fleeting, reliant on greying photos, story morsels that proffer jagged bits of information. I hold in my mind the image of a man, tall, handsome, intelligent, and at a space, a little way away a child, both encompassed by the shadow of polio.

Dr. Patricia Goldblatt is a former teacher of art and English in Toronto and program officer at the Ontario College of Teachers. She is the author and editor of two books on teaching as well as articles on women's issues, education, literature, and diversity. Her writing on travel has been published nationally.

Lie Down

Katherine Govier

As soon as I heard, I called Maxine. And she said, "If you want to join this death watch, you are welcome." I know it sounds bitter, but it wasn't really; it was just her vintage candor. I said, "I will come to visit. What can I bring?"

And Maxine said, *"An explanation."*

Of all the old friends, some will be reconciled, with or without a prognosis of death. Of all the dead, some will lie down and others will not. Maxine will not. After being given eighteen weeks and no hope, she lasted eighteen months in a remission so convincing that people took her for a liar. It was embarrassing because a wake had been planned. She was a terrific organizer, and this got organized right back at her. The date was set, and the invitations were out. They were raising money for a memorial award in her name. Maxine not only lived to attend her wake, looking fabulous, and gave a fine speech, but she has continued to live right through the next winter. She's pretty funny on the subject. Now when certain names come up she says, "Oh yeah, Bill gave money and now he's mad at me because I didn't die. He thinks I'm faking."

For a while it did appear that Maxine wasn't dying after all, at least not on that particular speeded-up schedule. She was offered a counsellor. But she emerged from the process claiming she'd been told she was doing so well in denial that she might as well stay there. We could be with her, but we couldn't have a say. We couldn't pity and we couldn't protest.

Maxine doesn't like being talked about and she doesn't like dying. I play by her rules, for now. Still, she won't escape either, much as she'd like to.

OUTSIDE a wind whips up the discarded donut wrappers and cigarette foil and makes them dance around tree trunks in front of the street-level window where I sit drinking coffee. A lot of sick people die just before the spring. They make it through the winter, but the warmth is so slow in coming they just wither.

People go by with their hands in their pockets and hair flying; they look in as if checking to see if I am real. For reasons not entirely within my control, the city is for me a fishbowl. I signal for the bill; passersby take note. I push back my chair carefully. It reminds me of a certain e.e. cummings poem where he says spring is the hand in the window moving things but not breaking anything. I can identify with window dressing.

I head down to her house. I'm going to take her out for lunch.

After that first call, I appeared, I brought a casserole. There was, however, no explanation for the fact we'd fallen out of touch. Maxine let me off the hook. "We don't need to talk about all that, do we?" she said. I listened instead.

Pretty well my favourite phrase—and this has nothing to do with Celine Dion—is, *It's all coming back to me*. You know that wonderful rush you get when some big lost chunk of your life swings back into view? Hearing Maxine's caustic voice brought back the following: 1975, feeling sophisticated, eating fettucine alfredo at Luigi's beside the Morrissey. Riding our bikes up Jarvis Street from our smart jobs in television. Discovering an actual outdoor café on Markham Street. Seeing Toronto Dance Theatre's nude males crawl out of black sacks on the lawn in front of Hart House. Always coming home to the third floor and calling the answering service for messages. Back then, there was no voice mail. This service was manned by out-of-work actors. "Hi there, did ya' have an okay day? A bunch of your friends called you," the star of tomorrow would say.

Maxine tells me that her tumour has reappeared (*all coming back to me*). The remission is over.

The news has made her angry. She insists, as she has before on occasion, that Rick, her ex-, gave her the cancer. She considers giving up. "A small sneaking part of me," she actually says, "welcomes the chance to lay down my responsibilities."

I listen. Once before, she admitted to me that she was frightened. Only once. We talk about Auschwitz, why do people carry on? Hope, she says. Hope of a last-minute rescue. And sometimes it comes.

When we first met, she'd had a miraculous recovery from a car accident. I walked into a party; she was there in two casts, propped up on pillows in a corner, with various men dancing attendance. While she was still on crutches we had meal after cheap meal on Bloor, at the Blue Cellar, exchanging intimacies. Her place on Palmerston was just a block over from mine. There was a schnitzel joint we called "the Hungarian"; the owner was a tuberous giant of a man who we were convinced was a Nazi war criminal. Once a year he stood on each of the little tables in his restaurant, one after another, hanging Christmas tinsel from the ceiling. It was a terrible thing to watch him climb on those spindly Formica numbers with screw-on aluminum legs. We feared the legs would give out, that he would topple, pulling down all the acoustic tiles into our breaded veal cutlets.

When people sink into illness their voices are the last thing to go. Hers is a bit raspy, surprisingly low for her tiny size. I could listen as long as she could talk. Certain remarks of hers, simple sentences uttered over nearly thirty years, stay with me as if the conversation took place only hours ago. "It was the real thing," she said of our friendship in a valedictory way when she considered our estrangement to be final. And, "You know I am on your side," once when a friend of hers made off with my serious lover. In the old days a group of us borrowed play sets from the Yorkville Library and did readings. I was always the ingenue. Maxine was the dowager.

"I guess you got that out of your system," I quipped on our last lunch.

She shot me a sharp glance. "I may have style, but I do not mean to make this look easy."

The dying are allowed to joke about it; we others are not.

FROM HER BEDSIDE, my eyes rove to the sunshine that I can see paving the normally grey street with a line of purest yellow. Spring is a perhaps hand in a window, the poet said, "carefully to and fro moving New and

Old Things." Which are we? Not new but not yet old, each spring a tad more faded, but we do have style; spry does not yet apply. We are light and loose, compared to the heavy furniture of the aged. Perhaps we always will be, we who live.

Although the hand does its stealthy damage. For instance, when did it arrange the free radicals and the cancer cells so delicately in Maxine's pancreas as to begin the slow destruction? No one saw. Perhaps for years no one knew. A year ago the disease blossomed; in summer it was mowed under; in winter it slept, and now with the season it wakes, ravenous.

She is tired. But she wants to come to lunch, so I help her dress. "Perhaps it's time to accept the inevitable," says Maxine, partway through getting the sweater on.

"Out of the question," I say. I put myself on the dream team from the start. "You'll see your fiftieth birthday," I say. "We're going to go to Mexico as soon as you're on your feet."

This too is a Toronto thing. Flight. I'm thinking I'll drive her down the highway that runs along the east coast. The A1A, it's called. It is a slow, two-lane highway that cars must share with bicycles. Driving, one is descended upon by flocks of aggressive cyclists with their lozenge-shaped, shiny, insect-like helmets. They swerve around you and curse and shake their fists so that you are glad air conditioning forces you to keep the windows rolled up.

I feel the lure of that road. When you get to the north of Florida you can turn off inland to Orlando. At Universal Studios there is a King Kong ride. An almost genial ape looms over the skyline and picks up the subway car you're riding in and threatens to peel it like a banana. Farther south the highway winds past the mansions of the very rich, and the stacked-up high-rise condominiums of the middle-class elder-folk who likewise flock there, and even past the trailer community of Briny Breezes, with its hair salon adorably called Briny Hair. The road is sometimes in sight of the beach, but more often the beach is hidden by wrought-iron gates, golf clubhouses, town bathing pavilions, and some of the few remaining natural dunes in the state. You can take this highway all the way to Miami, the Keys, to jump off for points south. I want to drive down it slowly, down, down to a place of easy long stupid days and no painful annual struggles to come back from the dead. Just me and Maxine and her intravenous.

WE SET OFF up the sidewalk, heading for Bloor Street and lunch. Maxine wears a morphine-dispensing box on her side that she punches when she feels pain, and a colostomy bag under her overalls. Her post-chemo hair is a khaki ruffle like the feathers on a baby chick. Her feet are so swollen she can't wear shoes: they are stuffed into a pair of clogs. She clings to my arm and stumbles. She looks down at her legs as she walks, and of course mine hove into view as well. "Your tights are navy," she says, "but you think they're black because you didn't look carefully."

At lunch she eats nothing. "You starve to death with this thing, that's what happens, did I tell you?" she says. She is so thin her spine stands out several inches from the flesh of her back and feels as hard as a row of nails. She wants me to touch it in the restaurant, just as, while she dressed, she wanted to show me the bag attached to her navel. She can't sit on chairs without cushions. In the sunlight I can see a fine white down on her face that is the same as the down my babies had when they were born, *lanugo*. When the morphine makes her lose the thread of the conversation she charges, "Bring me back!"

"Come back!" I say.

"I loved my body," she says.

I note the past tense.

She wants to talk about sex. She starts by telling me about a book written by a gay man, giving sex tips for women. "Don't bother with all that fancy stuff when you give a blow job," she says, "they just like it hard and deep." Her lover still climbs into bed with her; she needs to know that he desires her, that he is not put off by the bag of shit on her belly. Maxine avers that she has never been sure that men actually liked going down on women. But her lover now actually does. "It's a big mysterious organ, and making it move gives him a sense of power," she says.

I remember this sex talk from the seventies. Penis size, predilections, who lasted longer. It stopped for a couple of decades. But we are at it again. Marriage, loyalty to the fathers of our children, dropped the curtain of silence on this subject. It will take more than husbands to shut Maxine down. She can say what she wants. She is facing the distinguished thing, as Edith Wharton calls death, quoting Henry James.

When I take her home she is exhausted and lies on the bed. She thumps her morphine purse angrily until finally she slides into another place from which I do not bring her back. I look at her closed eyes and tell her how strong and brave she is and how our friendship is the real thing and that I am on her side.

As I leave she raises her eyelids. "Next time we'll go shopping to l'Elegance." That's a designer resale place on Yorkville. All her dresses are too big. She wants something smaller to be buried in. And will I take her for a facial and a body wax? Yes, I say. I'm pretty sure this will not happen. The nurse in charge of this campaign, Maxine's best—because we've arrived at the stage, finally, where people other than Maxine herself are in charge—will never allow it.

I walk downstairs and through her kitchen to the door. People are gathering, people who have been more consistent, people who never fell out, or who, I suppose, brought the explanations they were asked for. These custodians are talking about her fondly, marvelling at her every gesture and word, as if she is, as if she *were* a precocious child. I will not do it.

The wind whips my hair into my face as I say goodbye. I turn right and walk back up to Bloor. It happened while I was at her bedside; the wind took away the last of the cold. The half-concrete snow, the crust laced with black that lay along the curb so long this year, has vanished. Spring is so short here. By the time she's gone, a fine dust, the dust of summer, will be rising.

Katherine Govier has published nine novels, three short story collections, and two anthologies of travel writing. She has won the City of Toronto Book Award and the Marian Engel Award. Her novel Creation, *about John James Audubon, was a New York Times Notable Book of the Year. Her latest novel is* The Ghost Brush *(HarperCollins Canada). Katherine has been President of PEN Canada and Chair of the Writers' Trust. She helped establish both the student program Writers in Electronic Residence, and Canadian Journalism for Foreign Trained Writers, for refugee and immigrant writers.*

Friendship Bracelets

Jon Hunter

In Memory of Kenny

My daughter makes friendship bracelets. A skill learnt during the long car rides to the cottage as a way to pass the time, it was quickly forgotten when we arrived, and more active outdoorsy times beckoned.

But, over the years, sometimes on rainy days, sometimes as a break from the pressures of studying for exams, sometimes as a special gift for a friend or cousin, she would dig out the box of embroidery thread. Then you'd find her, crouched in the yard, or in front of the TV, bent over a skein of multi-coloured threads pinned to the knee of her jeans, twirling and knotting.

For awhile, I got one a summer. The process was always the same—a casual question as to whether I thought these colours went together well, then a few hours in that "native woman weaves cloth" pose, with intermittent "give me your wrist" demands. Eventually, on one of those occasions the bracelet would be deemed correct, and knotted around my wrist. Then, with a quick peck on the cheek, she'd move on to the next thing on her internal list of things to do. There was no clasp, no choice as to whether or not I wanted to wear it to work, for instance. That was the deal: I got it without asking, had only a little choice about how it looked, and even less about how long it lasted. But while it was there, it became a part of me, a perpetual reminder, just on the edge of consciousness, that somebody else cared enough about me to make this effort. The colours and design became perfect, because she picked them with me in mind and wanted me to have them.

Once I got it, it was tied on until the day when the cotton finally frayed enough to let go. No matter how ragged it became, its going almost always took me by surprise. I might have noticed a loose thread, or even retied the odd one, but when I awoke to find the bracelet loose in the bed, or felt an unexpected nakedness on my wrist in the middle of a busy day, I was always taken aback—a little sad, a little reluctant to give up the band of faded and blended tatters.

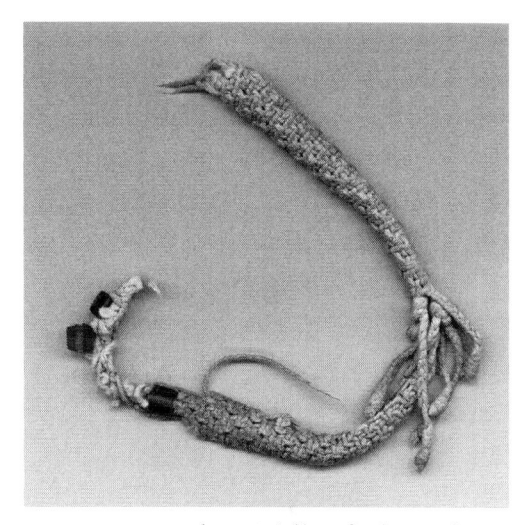

A short while ago a dear friend, someone I met during our training years ago, died. We saw each other's children grow, shared beefs and triumphs, and commiserated with each other over the big and the small— the worries about an ill child, or the haplessness of the Blue Jays. Our relationship was as unique as a friendship bracelet, woven at one moment in time, but bearing the signs of experience. In fact, it occurred to me that life is like this for any of us: We get a start; if we're lucky, it comes from a place of love. Then, once made, we begin to wear out. Our colours, once so distinct and clear, become melded into one another, more Monet than Mondrian. This change is not so much a loss of clarity as a development of character. Some threads break and are retied, others spray into a fan. Through it all, most of the time we pay it no heed; it is something that goes on while we concentrate on the things that feel immediate. We may have a dim awareness that it's not the same as it used to be, but we're used to having it, and feel no need to focus on it, at least, not right now. And then, the bracelet falls off. It hits us as if without warning, and even though the signs may have been there for some time, we are most often shocked.

For my friend, the signs came only a short time before he died, before his life was cut short, and he fell out of our lives, like a bracelet off a wrist. A bracelet too short-lived, but certainly one marked by generosity, love, and more than a bit of mischief in the design.

Some trace remains—as if the bracelet had left a white band on my wrist after a sunny summer. One can hope it will last forever.

Jon Hunter is an associate professor at the University of Toronto, and a staff psychiatrist at Mount Sinai Hospital, where he treats medically and surgically ill patients psychotherapeutically to help them with their adaptation to illness.

Hope from a Distance

Nigel Leaney

I've been at Julie's for only about half an hour when my mobile goes. The jaunty William Tell Overture gets louder in my pocket. It always reminds me of a couple shagging on fast forward. Julie sighs as I search my pocket. She already knows who it is. *Sam Calling*, it says. My fingers waver over the keypad before I take the call.

"Sam, is that you?"

"Hey, Jack, I'm sorry—I'm in a bit of trouble." Sam's voice is low and very soft. I have to strain to hear him.

"What's up, Sam? What trouble?"

"I'm down at the hospital. Please, can you help me?" Then I hear the voice of a female telling him that mobiles aren't allowed and the thing goes dead.

I look up at Julie. "I'm sorry, I have to go."

"No you don't *have* to, Jack, but, of course, I know you're going to."

"He's my brother. I have to try to help. You know that."

"And who am I? Who am I to you?" She pauses to soften her voice. "Please stay. We don't get these chances very often, a whole night together. Mick is back on days from tomorrow and we'll be back to sneaking around again."

"Like we're not sneaking around now?"

"You know what I mean."

I nod. Mick is a copper. Married to the job. Divorced from Julie in all but name. Anyway, that's the line I keep feeding myself to ease my conscience. "I still have to go."

The hospital is a short fifteen-minute drive. It's way past rush hour so traffic is light. I make an educated guess and head for A & E. It's a familiar route.

Sam lies abandoned in one of the cubicles. The curtains are only half drawn, so he is easy to find. He is on the bed staring up at the ceiling. Both of his wrists are heavily bandaged. How many stitches this time? I wonder.

"Hey, what happened?" I ask stupidly.

Sam doesn't reply. The ceiling is endlessly fascinating, I guess. I feel a sudden swell of anger but manage to hold it in check.

"Was it the voices again?" I continue.

Sam makes a grunt of affirmation that's barely audible.

"Sam, I'm here. Come on, turn and look at me." I keep my voice low and easy so he can't read the subtext: *I've busted my arse to get here, so the least you can do is turn round and talk to me properly, you selfish bastard.* No, I'm trained to stay closed and unreadable. But with Sam's keen sense of paranoia I'm never completely sure.

We stay for awhile fixed in time, a strange tableau framed by the curtains. Someone is screaming and cursing farther down the corridor. White coats flash by in the fast lane, tails billowing out. There's a cloying, clinical smell of disease and desperation.

"Looks like a fun night ahead," I say to no one but myself.

Sam remains motionless. I watch his chest rise and fall. Just breathing. Sometimes I wonder if he isn't right. If this is all life can bring him, then why bother? Do any of us know any better? But yet we keep patching him up, sending him off, telling him things will work out okay. But will they ever? Maybe he should just be allowed to do what he's been rehearsing for so long. Perhaps there's some nobility in suicide. My throat is dry, I start to feel hot. "I'm going to get a drink. I shan't be long. Can I get you anything?"

There's no response, so I leave. In the next building is a deserted canteen. Well, it's really just a vending machine with a few plastic chairs and tables scattered round. I sip the bitter coffee, wishing I'd gone for the chocolate.

Dr. Keeler told me how important it is not to get angry or overly critical. Keep a cool head at all times. Of course, that's easier said than done. And Keeler knows it, which is why he looked so uncomfortable, I guess. Both of us are sitting in his office with the sun streaming rudely through. How many times has he trotted out the same advice while fiddling with his gold nib fountain pen? But I'm not too bad. Really. At least I never show my frustrations to Sam. I keep them to myself, my smile stretched thin and tight. A face that stretches over the whole world with an eternal rage but always smiling, always hiding. And Sam, he's hiding too from voices that only he can hear. But it doesn't make them less real. There are three of them: tormentors that haunt him each day, sometimes loud, sometime whispers, but always malevolent. It seems his only escape would be death. But then that's what the voices want. That is their everlasting command. Every day it's the same, despite all the pills he takes. I can't imagine what it must be like and sit there in awe as my coffee cools.

I plunge back through the frames of the past, freezing onto Charlie Grant, and his fists waving above me. The cold, wet playground soaks slowly into my torn uniform. I taste blood. So this is what it's like. He steps back. I'm not sure whether it's to admire his own work or prepare for the good kicking. I'm aware of others standing by, flannel trousers, the bare legs of girls, all the spectators of my humiliation. It happens so fast it takes everyone by surprise. The thin crowd suddenly step back as he comes crashing through, Charlie Grant is still looking at me. He wants to takes his time over his moment of glory. First thing he is aware of is dropping to his knees and blood running down his chin. Then I see him. He stands between my assailant and me. Another punch and Charlie Grant is sprawled on the grey ground. He's not knocked out but he's not moving. His eyes are now fixed on Sam. I see real terror in them and I feel like laughing and singing. Sam helps me up, brushes me down, and we walk out the gates together, not saying anything, both fixed on the road ahead. Yes, that was Sam—my big brother.

So what happened? I was the young, nerdy one. The one with the bad stutter and crippling shyness. Mum gave me a sodalite crystal egg. She said it would help me to foster harmony and communication. That's one thing I loved about Mum. She was a real witch who diligently practised her Wiccan craft. And I guess it worked. I feel for the stone in my pocket and run my finger over its smooth surface. One small stone that I've carried in my pocket for around a decade. Between us we have plenty of mementos of her. But this stone is my one precious link. The one that counts. After the car crash and her death ten days later, was that when it all started? Can bereavement turn into madness?

Whatever, I think Sam had changed before that. A day before she died, Mum had asked me to look after him. He was already becoming part of community care. One of the state's vulnerable adults. Not much had been said about it. It was no big deal. He'd chalked up one short admission and regular trips to the surgery for his pills and a jab. Sam seemed to take even that in his stride for awhile. The real curtain callers came later. At least Mum was spared all that. And Dad? He hasn't featured for many years. Alive or dead, I neither know nor care.

I drain my coffee with a small shudder and make a slow return.

Sam has company. She straightens up as I approach and extends her hand over Sam. We shake. "Hi, I'm Kate. And you must be Jack, his brother."

I nod. "Are you a friend?"

"Sorry, I should have said. I'm a social worker from the Community Mental Health Team."

Despite her drooping eyes and white, drawn face, she doesn't look old enough. But lately that's a problem I've been having with a lot of people.

Kate is frowning. "Can we talk?"

I nod again, taking it to mean what it always does in these circumstances. She wants words away from Sam. We move a distance from the cubicle. I glance back with the guilt of a conspirator. But Sam is still staring up into another reality.

Kate gives me a searching look. I wonder how much she knows, being the out-of-hours social worker? Has she read his medical biography or is that what she wants from me?

"This isn't the first time," I say. A note of apology seeps through.

"And he's been on Section Three before?"

"Last year. It took a long time for him to get over it. And as you can see . . ." I trail off. What am I blathering about?

Kate stays locked on me; a heat-seeking missile, factual and emotionless. "The situation is this: Sam's was a serious attempt. And the way he's still presenting, he's certainly sectionable. Unless he'll go voluntarily, as an informal patient, do you think?"

I shake my head, hearing the cries and screams of last year. "Don't leave me here, Jack. Please don't." Had another male patient raped him? That's what he'd told me. But there was no evidence. I'd made noise and kicked up a fuss. But in the end they said it was part of his paranoid delusional system.

"So if that's the case," Kate continues, "I could get the duty consultant and GP to sign the necessary papers. It'll be for his own safety."

"You said *could*. Is there an alternative?"

Kate shrugs and turns slightly from me as if in momentary contemplation. "I rang round already and there is a problem with beds. Long View is full. There are no spaces, which would mean your brother would have to go to another hospital out of the area until a local bed becomes available. I'm not sure where else could take him, I'd have to do some more phoning around."

"He would hate that. I mean he hates Long View too. But this . . . this would be too much."

"That's why I wanted to talk to you."

"I don't know what to say. I mean what else . . . ?"

Kate rests her hand on my shoulder. "There's no rush. I imagine they'll want to keep him here overnight. Have a think about it." She glances at her watch. "Look, I'm sorry, but I need to be elsewhere. This is my number. Call me later. But I'll check in anyway just to see how things are."

She leaves me in an instant, stranded in the corridor. I stare back towards Sam's cubicle, stones filling up in my stomach. What am I supposed to be thinking about? Even then I still pretend to myself that I don't know, that there is no alternative to what she's just told me.

I sit by Sam's bed and wait, for what I don't know. He has no more lines in him. But he still looks phantom pale. And so thin.

Maybe it was all those drugs years ago. Tripping in the stone circle at Glastonbury Festival, waiting for the dawn to rise. Then the sun finally came, greeted by whoops and cheers and frenzied drumming from all the other dawn trippers. We'd done it all together. That and so much more. So why is it not me lying there too?

I begin to get sleepy. Resting my eyes, my neck keeps flopping down, then jerks me awake. I slump lower in the chair to support my neck and drop into a state of half sleep. Hours must have passed. I suddenly feel rough crepe against my skin and a hand groping for mine. "Get me out of here," Sam whispers.

I turn to look into his petrified eyes and pat his now limp hand. "It's okay, Sam. It'll be okay. You've got me. Just give me one minute and I'll be back."

I stand outside on the steps of the hospital. There's a thin light. Dawn is about to break. I turn on my mobile to make two calls. The first is to Julie, which is answered by her voicemail. I knew it would be. I could have waited until a more reasonable hour when she'd have picked up, but this was my coward's way out. I'm not ending our relationship exactly, but I know she won't understand my decision. So it won't survive, not this time. Then I dial Kate's number, who answers as brightly as the hour permits.

She listens carefully to what I say; all I can hear is her slight breath. I imagine her going through the risk assessment as I speak. Not that I blame her.

"Okay," she says, "but I'll need to hand this over to my colleagues in the morning. But don't worry. We may just need to visit. It's now as much about you as Sam. You may be glad of some support."

"Well, we'll see how it goes," I say lamely. "Thanks anyway."

"Don't thank me," Kate says and leaves the rest unsaid. I guess I was about to save the local authority a whole bundle in out-of-area costs. Not to mention all the hassle and paperwork.

When I return to Sam, he's sitting up and mumbling something to one of the nurses.

"Can he go soon?" I ask her.

"I think so. The doctor will want to take one final look at him before discharge, but it won't be long."

"Can I take him outside for some air?"

She nods cautiously. "But not too long."

We sit on the steps outside and share a cigarette. I find the sodalite crystal in my pocket and hold its egg shape up to the dawn light.

"Remember this?"

Sam frowns. I drop the egg in his hand.

"It's yours now. It's done all it can for me. Mum wants this for you now."

Sam examines the crystal in his hand, studying its lines; imperfections and the way the light of a new day makes it glow slightly with a blue luminescence. Without a word he slips it into his pocket. The silence is awkward. An event has passed between us that neither of us is ready to recognise yet.

"Come on, " I say. "Let's go see the doc and get you out of here."

"W-w-where?" Sam asks.

I look at him with mock incredulity.

"My place, of course. We're together now. That's if it's okay with you?"

And for the first time in a long while I see a ghost of a smile slide across Sam's face.

Nigel Leaney is a mental health nurse with a BA and BSc in psycho-social interventions in psychosis. He also writes a regular column for a U.K. social work magazine and has won prizes for short fiction.

Something Happened

Jane Martin

For Ewen McCuaig (1931–2001)

> Sor Juana, do you not think this might be the singular gift of women's art? To ennoble yearning, and imbue it with a kind of grace?
> —The Viscount, *Hunger's Bride,* Paul Anderson

The titles of the exhibition and the drawings in it are taken from things Ewen said. The changes in Ewen's language represent not so much a change as an intensification of his perception. A few of his expressions were funny, although not to him, some very concrete, others original, magical, and profound. Everything he said seemed momentous.

Very rapidly over Thanksgiving weekend 2000 Ewen's memory fell by the wayside. Floating on his back in the swimming pool, he saw every detail of the ceiling with excruciating clarity without being able to figure out where he was. I thought he was having a stroke. After many hours at the emergency department we were told that he was not having a stroke and to go home. At dinner that night I asked Ewen to talk to me about what he thought was wrong. He raised his hand slowly, lightly touched his left temple, and said quietly, *"Something happened to my brain."*

Back in the hospital some days later, Ewen was so afraid of forgetting my name he wrote it on a scrap of paper and placed it on his over-the-bed table so he would be ready if "they" asked him what his wife's name was. Of the MRI, he said, *"There was this noise thing and then I lost everything."*

After his surgery, trying to make a little joke, I looked at Ewen's helmet and asked him if they'd shaved his hair. He raised his hands close to his helmet-covered ears and said, "Oh no, I have hair. *I can hear it tick."*

Later he corrected himself and said that they had cut the grass but they told him, "*The grass grows back.*" Explaining the surgery to me two days later Ewen said, "*What grew in there by false, the stone, is removed. They throw away the stone. We have no idea the quantity at home.*"

Ewen awoke the morning after his surgery and said, "*I'm so sad overnight thinking of the policeman who died at forty-five.*" I was struck that his sadness was for a stranger and not for himself. For the rest of his days Ewen remained what he had always been: devoid of self-pity and full of empathy for others. He looked forward to "*All the lovely things I have to do.*"

Barry and James, who lived with us then, had a huge bunch of roses waiting for us when we got home. As the roses opened over the next few days, Ewen exclaimed, "*The roses were just moving into fabulosity.*" The following June the hundreds of blooms in the rose gardens at 21 Rose Avenue were fabulosity itself.

On the August holiday weekend, Ewen was back in the hospital. A coloured square was drawn on his chest to guide the radiation machine. I worried when I inadvertently washed off some of this green drawing, but the technician said it didn't matter as the marks were tattooed in. As it happened, we had a young niece and her friend staying with us who then wanted to show Ewen their tattoos.

Ewen continued to swim for the rest of his life. Water became the only place he could move painlessly and with a sense of freedom. The bathtub too was "*the swimming place.*" He loved being at the cottage and lying in "*the hanging bed*"—a name I now prefer to "hammock."

What amazed me was how Ewen, feeling his "*whole body in devastation, time flying by so fast,*" and close to leaving "*all the lovely things I have to do*" undone, could still find "*there are questions I don't know the answer to,*" could say, "*Though I accepted what happened, this is almost like a miracle . . . all the energy,*" state, "*For me this place is like a revelation,*" could "*feel that thing coming over my heart in waves,*" and wonder "*if there's another place nearby where things are different.*"

Something Happened: Do Not Fail to Pay Attention is based on a photo I took of Ewen on 17 November 2001, a week before his death and the day he left 21 Rose Avenue for the last time. He said, not in any context but quietly into the air, "*Do not fail to pay attention.*" He didn't mean that we shouldn't fail to pay attention to him. He meant, Do not fail to pay attention to life, to love, to our medical system, and to this terrible disease. This work is my "paying attention."

Jane Martin is a senior Canadian artist whose work is in the permanent collections of public galleries from coast to coast, including the National Gallery of Canada and the Art Gallery of Ontario.

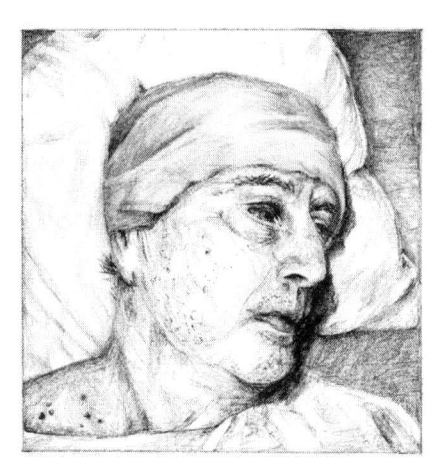

Something Happened: This Noise Thing and Then I Lost Everything. 11 x 9 cm. Pencil and coloured pencil. Coll. Erna Paris and Tom Robinson. © CARCC.

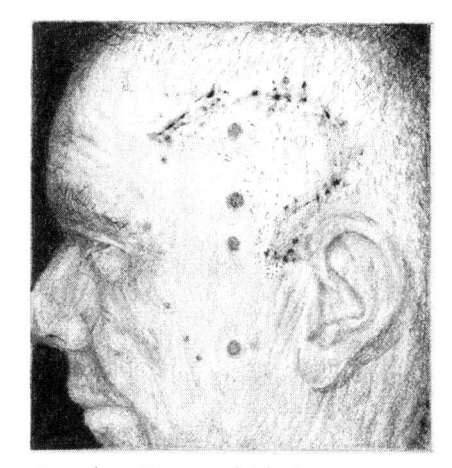

Something Happened: The Roses Are Just Moving into Fabulosity. 11 x 9 cm. Pencil and coloured pencil. Coll. Daintry Topshee. © CARCC.

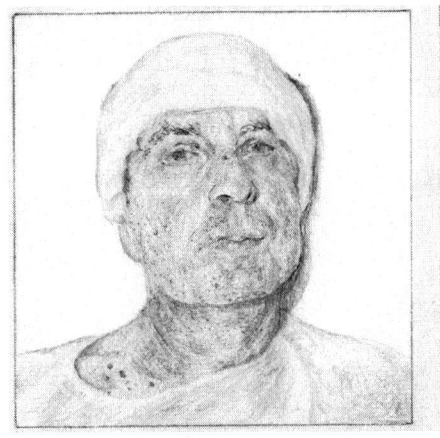

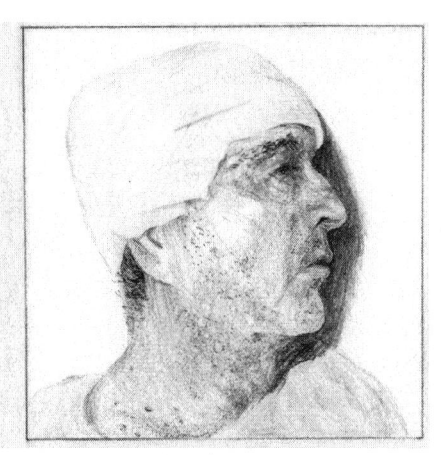

Something Happened: I Can Hear It Tick #1. 11 x 18 cm. Pencil and coloured pencil. Coll. Erna Paris and Tom Robinson. © CARCC.

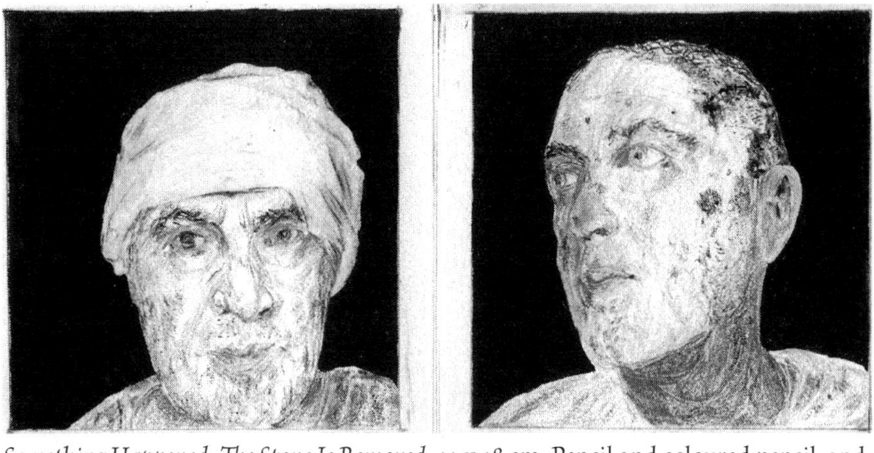

Something Happened: The Stone Is Removed. 11 x 18 cm. Pencil and coloured pencil, and watercolour. Coll. Art Gallery of Ontario by John McKinven and Bill Brown. © CARCC.

The Right Thing to Say

Kathy Page

Beneath a fierce September sky, the city squats in the ochre plain: a cluster of rectangular towers, surrounded by a vast, ever-growing sprawl of homes and stores. Don is driving Marla's car, the Corolla, which he cleaned out yesterday and filled with gas, to save them having to think about it today. He slows to fifty as he passes Safeway.

"Nearly there," he says, patting her leg, and she nods.

"Music, love?" he asks; this time she shakes her head.

She's sitting there looking straight ahead as they sail past dusty motels, a gas station, the ski rental. She wears sunglasses; her hands are folded in her lap. No sign of the baby yet, of course. A stranger wouldn't know what she's going through. Usually she's the one who knows what to say, who wants everything put into words, but now she's fallen silent, and really, Don thinks, there probably is nothing that they haven't talked over twenty or two hundred times already. In a few minutes they will have an answer: it just better be the one they want, OK, Whoever-You-Are-Up-There?

Fifty-fifty. Whichever way you peer at it, it's the same. Quite big. If you had a fifty-fifty chance of winning the lottery, you'd be pretty much on the edge of your seat. It's kind of the opposite of that, multiplied.

This morning Marla dressed to make a show of strength: denim skirt, fitted, lace-trimmed blouse, jewellery—all new things he hasn't seen before. Don went the other way and now he'd like to be able to say something, to find the right words. But instead, his mind is full of dumb, trivial thoughts, such as, It's a holiday, and it's lunchtime. They could be grilling some chicken on the barbecue. What was in that marinade they used last time? He glances across at Marla again and almost asks but stops himself.

They could be hiking, or gliding along the Kananaskis in their kayaks. But instead, because Dr. Ludvigssen has decided to go on vacation tomorrow, when every other person is returning, they're going for results.

"I can't wait another month," she said. Her call.

Don waits for three Lycra-clad cyclists to waver across the crosswalk, going towards the park.

After this, he thinks, he'll definitely sign up at the gym. Not that Marla has ever complained, and he is probably fitter than he looks, given his work. But something else is needed to pull it all together.

Crushed juniper berries, he remembers. Honey. Red wine.

The hospital blocks come into sight on the right-hand side: a huge place. Every kind of specialist you could ever not want to have to see.

"DO YOU HAVE a gut feeling for what your result will be?" Dr. MacLeod, the psychiatrist, asked, weeks ago in one of the early consultations.

"Yes," Marla said, "it's silly, I know, but I don't want to say it."

"Me?" Don said, "Marla is fine. Has to be. That's what I feel."

"The trouble with gut feelings," Dr. MacLeod said in that voice of his, subdued, but insistent, "is that they have absolutely no bearing on the facts. Studies show that people are wrong as often as they are right. Suppose your gut feeling was wrong?" he said. "I'm just asking you both to consider that, in the intervening time."

I am not wrong, Don thought.

But now, with Marla stately and silent beside him as he drives towards the answer that has always been in her body, written, as the genetic counsellor explained it, in the paired genes of chromosome number four, his hands sweat against the wheel.

Because they don't need to do this. They could leave the answer in its sealed envelope, turn right around, and drive back towards the mountains, go home, eat, make love, soak together in the tub, doze, dream, continue from tomorrow as before. The baby's risk is only half of Marla's. Just 25 per cent! They can just keep their fingers crossed, live for the moment, the way they have so far—

"Lights!" Marla yells. He jams his foot down and the seatbelts lock, biting into their shoulders; their heads thud into the headrests. There is a blissful moment of nothing at all, followed by the blare of a horn. He's way over the line and in the wrong lane too.

"Are you OK?"

"I think so," she says. "You?"

"Sorry, sorry," he says, pulling air into his lungs. Everything is brighter than it used to be. "It wasn't the idea to total us on the way! Or give us heart attacks. Mind you, we're convenient for Emergency!"

"True." Her lips twitch. "It's green, now."

HE CHECKS, double checks, takes the right, then the next right. The hospital complex, oddly still, swallows them. Parkade 6 is almost empty. He switches off, leans back in his seat, turns to look at her.

"And we're ten minutes early," he says.

"We may as well go in. I can use the washroom."

I don't want to go in, he thinks, not until we have to.

WHEN SHE TAKES her sunglasses off and kisses him on the lips, her mouth is hot and tastes of mint.

Maybe, he thinks, she'll change her mind about this, even now?

BUT SHE CLIMBS out of the car and he follows her. Again, he badly wants to say something. The right thing. Not just *I love you*. Something more like *I'm with you. And if it's*—

It won't be.

"Marla—" is what he manages, as the entrance doors slide apart. He follows her into the elevator, out again.

The place is deserted: no receptionist, no bustle of file-wielding people passing through, and no sick people on the row of grey chairs and that, he thinks, is a relief. It's ten past one.

"They'll be here soon," she says. "I won't be long." He watches her until she turns the corner, then eases into one of the chairs and finds himself facing the leaflet rack, where, he knows, innocent-looking booklets and concertina-folded sheets of paper harbour phrases such as, "This is a late-onset, inherited brain disorder that causes progressive deterioration of the physical, cognitive, and emotional self."

How does she keep herself together the way she does, with this hanging over her? She has her mantra, of course: Even If, she calls it. Even if I do have it, I feel fine now. Even if, it might not show for another ten years . . . that kind of thing. She has her mantra, and then she can make a joke about almost anything, and she keeps very busy. Marla does not waste her time.

Don digs his fingers into his palms and squeezes his eyes shut.

He thinks of Marla as he saw her once, quite early on, when she had car trouble and he went to collect her from the school at the end of the day. He could have waited in the car but he sat on one of the benches outside the classroom and watched her through the glass panel in the door as she pointed to a list on the board, asked a question, then said something that sent the class laughing. It was strange and wonderful to see her like this, dressed in a rather sober fashion, doing things that would be impossible for him. A minute later, she opened the door, a sea of waist-high students churning behind her, and noticed him.

"No one leaves until you're quieter," she said to the class, and then, to him, pointing, mock solemn, "I'll see you later, Don."

"Yes, Miss."

SHE WAS ALWAYS CLEAR. She told him about it on their third date, and a few months later at Christmas he went with her to visit her mother. He had seen how she was.

At their wedding, Don remembers, they stood next to each other in the shade, facing the guests, and repeated their vows after the registrar. There was a script. They took turns. He felt her beside him, the body he knew so well cased in its strange, elaborate dress. His voice came out loud and clear and, despite the preceding weeks of jokes with friends about "needing to be committed," he felt absolutely sure. He promised there would be no others. He promised to be with Marla in sickness or in health and certainly, by then, he thought he knew what he was promising.

The wedding was in July, on Ed Wagner's ranch. All the fields were baled and beyond them you could see the mountains rearing up, purple grey, and some clouds boiling yet further above.

Her father said they deserved the best of everything in life and raised a glass. His father made a rambling speech about Marla's brains and

Don's hands and how at least they'd always have a roof over their head, a table to eat at, and never be short of conversation, and she cupped a hand to his ear and whispered that hands were all very well but there were other things he had about him too—and guests who saw the whisper somehow guessed what she was saying, banged on the table and roared.

BUT HERE'S THE THING: Despite everything she said, despite the recent assault course of leaflets, video, psychiatrist, counsellor, neurologist—despite all their best efforts and his own, despite *thinking* he had taken it on, he has never really been able to *imagine* that someone might actually dare to say to Marla, "You have it, too." He's listened, he's looked, but he has never believed, not even for moment or two until now, here in the Foothills Hospital's deserted waiting room, where he sits in a kind of vertigo, driving his nails into his palms and asking himself, What if there *is* bad news? How will I be for her? What will I do, what will I say to her as she turns to me? And what will I find myself feeling?

When you say *I do*, even to sickness and health, you're not thinking exactly of this. Will he know the right things to do and be able to do them? Be able to bear it, to change himself into what is needed—or, will he run, as Marla's father did (and no one, not even Marla, really blamed the man).

At work, he gets the instructions or drawings, sees what's required. He lines up the materials and tools, begins where it has to be begun, and works his way through. Measure twice, cut once. So long as your attention is on the job, it works out. But this is not the same. He doesn't know.

And now it's one fifteen, and a tall woman in loose, elegant clothes is walking towards him.

"Don. I'm Juliette." He remembers her from the first appointment. Warm hands, soft voice, a way of being able to look you in the eye without staring. He likes her.

"She's in the washroom," he says, just as Marla appears. His heart gears up as she stands next to him and reaches for his hand.

"Here we are, then," Juliette says, looking at each of them in turn. "We can go ahead now, but of course, if you're having any kind of misgivings, you do know we can put a hold on this."

"I want to go ahead," Marla says. Juliette nods.

"I'll call Dr. Ludvigssen and tell her you're here." As she walks to reception and picks up the phone, Don and Marla turn in to each other and embrace, their hands gripping hard, squeezing themselves against each other, their minds emptied out.

"THIS WAY." Marla follows, then Don. A left, a right, two lefts, right again.

When they came before, it was full of people, even in the corridors.

Now, there's just a faint rustle of clothes, their own muffled footsteps, the building's permanent hum. Names on the doors with strings of letters after them. FRCPC. FCCMG.

THE DOOR marked Dr. Ludvigssen is half open. There's a desk, two chairs, and an examining couch on the wall opposite the desk. A pink-cheeked woman with a shock of almost white hair is standing behind her desk. She clasps each of their hands, waves them into their chairs, and sits down as they do so. How was their journey over?

Come on! Don thinks, as Marla explains that the drive was a little tense. Hurry! he orders the doctor in his head.

"I shan't keep you waiting. I have your lab report here, Marla," Dr. Ludvigssen says. There's not enough space in the room. Not enough air, either, Don thinks, Marla's hand in his, damp, hot. Suddenly, now, it's all going too fast. The doctor slips her paperknife into the corner of the envelope and draws it across. She replaces the knife in her desk drawer, extracts and unfolds the letter, flattens it on the desk, and leans over it. Marla closes her eyes; Don, though, watches the doctor scan the page. Her face is very still, mask-like. There's a kind of high-pitched ringing in his ears, a feeling of imminent explosion in his chest and then, the moment before she speaks, he sees the corners of her eyes and mouth relax.

"It's good news," she says, and Don's on his feet with no idea how he got there.

"Marla!" She looks up at him, her face as he has never seen it before: eyes startled wide, her mouth a perfect O.

"Are you sure?" she asks, turning back to Dr. Ludvigssen.

"Yes. Your results are well within the normal range." Don pulls his chair closer, sits down again with his arm tight around Marla's shoulders as Dr. Ludvigssen continues, speaking slowly, nodding and smiling as she goes. When she uses the word "unambiguous," she corrects herself and says "completely clear." She turns around the report from the lab so that they can read it from their side of the desk. Her finger points to numbers and abbreviations, to a line of wave forms wiggling across the page—pretty much incomprehensible to a finishing carpenter, or for that matter an elementary school teacher, but everything is all right. The piece of code that unpicked Marla's mother has not been handed down, and that is the end of it.

Marla wipes her eyes and leans back in her chair. One of her arms is flung out to the side.

"Thank you both so much," she says. Dr. Ludvigssen glances at Juliette, smiles.

"I'm very pleased for you," she says, "But I have to say we can't take the credit there. Good or bad, we don't make these results and nor does the lab. We just bring the news."

"Well," Marla insists, "thank you for that. For coming in today." Everyone smiles and nods and then Juliette says that even when they have fantastic news like this, people do sometimes have unexpected reactions, so please do get in touch if that happens or they need anything or with any questions—otherwise, she will call in a month or so.

She stands, the doctor follows suit. Hands are shaken. It's over. Yet something keeps Don in his chair.

"Why not stay here awhile?" Juliette suggests. "It's really not a good idea to drive straight away. Leave when you're ready."

"Enjoy your holiday!" Don tells Dr. Ludvigssen.

How often, he thinks, do those two have to go through this?

THEY'RE ALONE. A breath of outside air pushes at the blind, shifting the light in the room and making a faint clattering noise. The room and everything in it—the poster about neurons above the examining table, the blue mug on the bookshelf, the film of dust on the blinds, the dead plant on Dr. Ludvigssen's desk—all of it seems alert, almost alive. Even the air is different, charged and delicious. They breathe deeply, filling themselves up. They turn the chairs face on so that they can absorb each other with their eyes.

She's smiling, and her face still has some of that shocked-open look. She looks different. Younger. Her old self but a new one at the same time. She chuckles, points to the withered plant on Dr. Ludvigssen's desk.

"I bet someone gave her that!" Hearing her laugh, Don starts to cry.

"Hey," Marla says, still smiling. He can't smile back. Mouth, throat, lips—all of them seem to have a will of their own and none of them want to coordinate.

"The thing is—" he wipes his face on his arms, tries again. "This is really fucking dumb," he manages to say, taking her hands in his. "This is not the right thing to say. But—see—I won't know, Marla. I'll never know how I would have been for you."

They stand and she pulls him to her, tight, his head on her shoulder, his tears making her blouse wet, like he's never going to stop.

Kathy Page is the author of seven novels, including Alphabet, *nominated for a Governor General's Award. Her interest in how we construe knowledge about our medical futures is further developed in* The Find, *forthcoming.*

Second Round

Nancy Richler

Like most desertions, it was unexpected. Gina awoke one morning to find her looks gone. Vanished. Replaced by a moonscape of enlarged pores, webs of pink veins, and discoloured pouches under her eyes. She was thirty-nine.

She had thought she was prepared, had already started watching for the thinning of the skin around her eyes, the softening of her jawline, the appearance of a fine, then coarse network of wrinkles and creases as her face folded itself permanently along the lines of her moods and personality. She had planned to be graceful about it, to accept the natural course of things, but this she hadn't expected. The suddenness of it, the ruthlessness—as if the hand of time had struck her one hard right across the face as she had slept undefended.

"Make-up covers a multitude of sins." She could hear her mother's voice as she studied the damaged reflection. What she faced, though, seemed less a sin than a disaster area, a battlefield on which a war of attrition was being waged. She touched the skin under her eyes, lightly, gingerly, afraid it might break under her fingertip. It sprang back, purple, but still alive. She reached for the concealer cream, remembered she'd run out, and made a mental note to pick some up on her way home from work. Then she remembered she wasn't going to work that day.

She went to the kitchen to make tea. She never had breakfast the mornings of Sandra's chemo, but drank tea instead, cup after cup of clear tea, until it was time to go to the hospital. As she poured her third cup she noticed a crack running down the length of the teapot. A fine long crack, just deep enough to allow the lead from the clay beneath the enamel to seep into the brewing tea.

She poured the rest of her tea down the sink and went back to her bedroom to get dressed. She always took extra care with her appearance on the days she had to go to the hospital. Faced with her reflection again, she closed her eyes. She pressed a hot washcloth against the discoloured pouches, then scrubbed lightly around the edges of her nose, taking care not to irritate the new webs of pink capillaries.

Her life hadn't prepared her for the demands it would make, she decided, not for the first time. Maybe no one's did, but she felt uniquely unprepared. "Spoiled" was how her ex-husband had put it soon after their wedding. Humiliatingly soon. Until then she had simply thought herself well loved. (My three jewels is what her father called her and her sisters, pleased and proud that his daughters were so pretty. And so lively—he had never liked morose women.)

"Happy enough," is what she told her sisters about her marriage after that, even after Pete's eye began to wander. "Happier than nothing," she changed her report when the rest of him wandered too. Would she and Pete have remained that way—happier than nothing—she wondered now? Would that have been the defining statement of her life when all was said and done? Happier than nothing?

Armchair questions, she decided. One of Pete's other women had gotten pregnant. Gotten pregnant and decided she wanted to keep the baby. Decided she wanted to keep the father too.

"Phillipa!" Sandra spat when Gina told her what was happening. "I've always hated pretentious names."

"It's not pretentious, it's English," Gina said. ("What's she like?" she'd asked Pete, imagining a cool, grey-eyed blonde. "I don't know," Pete shrugged. "Full of life," he said, managing to hit Gina twice with one statement.)

Their older sister Debra took Gina's hand. "What are you going to do?"

"*I'm* not going to do anything. *He's* going to leave me."

"You should get a job," Pete suggested when he was over one night dividing the books. They had just flipped a coin over a hard-covered copy of *Tale of Two Cities*, which was now sitting on Pete's pile, and were moving on to *The Prophet*—which Gina was prepared to fight for—when Pete asked how she was doing. She responded by bursting into tears. "OK, I guess, all things considered." That's when Pete made the suggestion about the job.

"You're a smart woman, Gina. There's no reason for you to spend the rest of your life turning into your mother."

Gina stared at him, stunned for a moment.

"My mother has a husband and three daughters who adore her," she said quietly. It had been her fondest wish that she could turn out like her.

Gina did get a job shortly after that, as a receptionist at a veterinarian's. She found it difficult work.

"There's something about the dogs' lack of wariness when they first come in," she told Sandra one evening when they met for coffee. "That pathetically optimistic tail wagging. Not all the dogs, of course, but there was a spaniel this morning that was in for surgery, pretty major surgery . . ."

Sandra wasn't listening. She put down the coffee cup she'd been holding in front of her face and revealed that she and Paul had been trying to have a baby and she wasn't conceiving. "And now they want to send me for tests," she burst out.

Gina tried to reassure her that everything would work out fine, but they both knew that Gina had had the very same problem. She'd tried for years to get pregnant. Right up until the moment that Pete had told her Phillipa was full of life. "I'm sure it will turn out differently for you," Gina said. And it had.

At first they had hoped it was a mistake. Sandra was the youngest of the sisters, the prettiest, the liveliest. It had to be a mistake. Each time the phone rang in Sandra and Paul's kitchen, one of them would run to answer, hoping it was the hospital calling to say there'd been a mix-up, that one of the technicians had mistakenly attached Sandra's name to another woman's tumour. The hospital would apologize and the family would be forgiving, grateful for the second chance Sandra had been given.

But the calls that came from the hospital weren't about mistaken diagnoses. They were about pre-operative procedures and scheduling surgery. And the second chance that Sandra was given didn't come from some lab technician's mistake. It came from the chemical mixture they dripped into her arm for the next six months. And it lasted only a year and a half.

At 8:30 Gina called Sandra to see if she was ready to go. Paul said she was already waiting outside. When Gina rounded the corner she could see

Sandra standing alone on the sidewalk, her fuchsia coat the only splash of colour on the November street.

"New coat?" Gina asked as Sandra slid in beside her.

"I'm not sure about the colour."

The colour was ghastly, grotesque even, against skin that had taken on such a yellow hue.

"I ran into Pete yesterday," Gina said, to change the subject.

"And?"

"Phillipa had another girl."

"When?" Sandra asked.

"Just last week. Apparently she has Pete's chin." Gina was about to joke that the chin was God's way of punishing, but then she didn't. Punishing who? Pete and Phillipa? The baby? And for what? And was that why things happened to people anyway, to reward and punish? This was the way Gina's thoughts worked lately. She knew it was morose.

Their mother was waiting outside her apartment building. As was Debra. "Nice coat," Debra said, giving Sandra's shoulder a squeeze. "Only you could pull off a colour like that."

The waiting room was fuller than usual. Many of the faces were familiar, but there were a few new ones as well. There were always a few new ones. "Cancer is a growth industry," Sandra had whispered once, setting off a round of giggles, which they had tried to control, but couldn't. As they stood at the entrance to the waiting room their mother motioned to Sandra to take the one vacant seat.

"You take it, Ma. I'll have time enough later to sit."

"No, you sit, Sandra," their mother insisted.

To cut the argument short, Debra took the seat. It was between two patients who always came on the same days as Sandra. Both liked to pass the time before their appointment by talking about their treatments, which was why Sandra didn't want to sit there. Sandra wasn't interested in her treatment anymore. It had been obvious for a while, though no one had mentioned it yet.

"I'd rather learn to fly," Sandra had said, finally, just that morning on their drive to the hospital.

"You always were a daredevil," Gina had responded, horrified to hear anger creeping into her voice.

"I dream about it a lot," Sandra said. "It's the same dream always: the earth, this incredible vivid green, falling fast and far beneath me."

In the rear-view mirror, Gina saw her mother's eyes.

Can't you ever think of anyone's feelings but your own? Gina almost burst out at Sandra. Sandra had always been the most self-centred of the sisters.

"You know we'll help you do anything you want to," Debra said quietly.

So Debra took the empty seat in the waiting room and heard about the nagging metallic taste in the man's mouth and the unusual fatigue the woman had experienced a whole five days after the last treatment. Debra recommended to the man that he try drinking peppermint tea, which he thanked her for as sincerely as if she'd suggested something that might help.

"There's another seat, Sandra," their mother said.

"You take it, Ma. Really, I'm fine."

Gina knew that their mother wouldn't take the seat while Sandra remained standing. There was nothing she could do about Sandra's lost hair or the nausea that overwhelmed her for days after each treatment, but she could at least remain standing by the entrance of the waiting room for as long as Sandra did. Gina took the vacant seat and waited for the nurse to call them.

The first time around they had all concentrated very hard during the treatments. Sandra had believed that it was important to imagine the chemicals entering her body, travelling to the farthest reaches, seeking out every last cancer cell and killing it. She'd kept her eyes closed the whole time the drip was in her arm, and whoever was with her closed her eyes too, adding her own focused concentration to the arsenal. This time, though, Sandra wanted to be distracted.

"How's the zoo?" she asked Gina as she lay down and offered the nurse her arm.

"Good. Fine," Gina said. She was actually amazed at how much she was beginning to enjoy the work. She had even recently begun thinking about applying to vet school, but it seemed tactless to say something like that to Sandra. Callous. "My allergies aren't bothering me in the least."

"Since when do you have allergies?"

The nurse cut in with a story about how she'd cured herself of a horse allergy years earlier by a mixture of diet and positive thinking. It was the type of story Gina didn't like. People were always telling Sandra stories about how other people cured themselves of everything from warts to brain tumours by thinking positive thoughts or eating food that no normal person would want to think about putting into her mouth.

Gina looked beyond Sandra to the window so she wouldn't have to see the last vial emptying into Sandra's arm. The tree outside the window had been in bloom when they'd started coming. A huge old chestnut, it was bare now. When Sandra finished this round, tight buds would be beginning to form again. The nurse finished her story just as she was ready to pull the needle out.

"You know what Debra said in the car?" Sandra asked Gina. "About helping me do whatever it is I want to do?"

"You're supposed to be resting," Gina reminded her.

Sandra was quiet for a few moments, then asked Gina if she'd seen *La Comtesse de Baton Rouge*. "Paul and I rented it last night. There's a character in it who's a human cannon. It's the coolest thing. She just climbs into the cannon, someone lights the fuse, then *wham*." Sandra's arm shot out from her body. "Can you imagine the rush?"

Gina knew some response was required of her, some acknowledgement that every word of Sandra's mouth now seemed to involve hurtling away from the earth at high speeds. All she could think of was the first time she had ever seen Sandra, all wrapped up in a pink blanket so only her little red face was showing. She reached for Sandra's hand. Sandra shut her eyes.

"Dad was holding you the first time I saw you," Gina said.

"Was I cute?"

"Not really. I'd been expecting you to be like a little doll, but . . ."

Sandra smiled. "That bad?"

"No. Not bad. It's just . . . I didn't expect you to be . . . real."

Sandra nodded, her eyes still closed.

"Who lit the fuse?" Gina asked. "In the movie."

Sandra thought for a minute. "I'm not sure." She smiled again and looked at Gina. "Not her sister."

Sandra held onto Gina as they walked back down the hall. She wanted to splash a bit of water on her face, so Gina went with her into the bathroom to splash some water on her own. The same face that had greeted Gina that morning stared back at her now. Beside her, Sandra washed her own face, which, at thirty-three, still looked young, despite the yellowish cast.

As Sandra started reapplying her make-up, Gina splashed some more water on her face. She had a quick flash of the waiting room on the evening after Sandra's second surgery. Their mother pulling at the hair around her temples, their father trying to soothe her with words too soft for Gina to hear. And Gina knowing in that instant that she'd never experience what it is to love or lose a child of her own.

"Ready to go?" she asked Sandra.

"Just one sec," Sandra answered, dabbing a bit more colour on a face that would never lose itself to the sorrows and relief of middle age.

Nancy Richler lives in Vancouver. Her most recent novel, Your Mouth Is Lovely, *was published by HarperCollins in 2002, and won the 2003 Canadian Jewish Book Award and Italy's 2004 Adei Wizo Award.*

On Different Hospital Floors

Nicholas Samaras

James, Two Days Old
How could I leave him, even
as his parents had left him
to go home and sleep?

In what imaginable world
could a mother inhale white lines
in her ninth month—her ninth month—
inducing instant labour and James
to be born brain-dead and twitching?

How could I leave him, even
as I lifted his perfectly-formed body
in the emergency air of baptism, even
as I whispered myself his godfather
and breathed his brief name for him,
and rocked him in a hospital room
abandoned of family,
whispering to him for hours,
even as I listened
for his breathing
and held his tiny dying
in my arms?

Ghazal as One Breath Holding

The Intensive Care nurse was neutral: all he has to do is take one day,
	each breath
at a time. I looked past her to my heart. What did she say? Did she say
	each breath?

My heart, my father on the monitor. Papa, you are all of these parts:
	your massive
chest, the mossy breasts, the warmth of my childhood. Hear it: one day,
	each breath.

Live through this. Past the bypass surgery, the harvesting of femur veins.
	Oh, Father,
I inhaled and held my sides, as I watched your chest narrow and splay to
	each breath.

The hesitations of your ribs grew longer, its cage heavier to lift. I watched
	you where
petition is the murmur of warmed-over air, where prayer is but the play
	of each breath.

And what can I tell my unborn children, about their grandfather who
	struggled for time
to see them? I implored the Mother of God, the Lord. Give him, I
	prayed, each breath.

One more breath. Papa, I held on for you. The tired staff went home.
	Into morning,
I held your hands in this world. I lived my life in that moment, so grey
	each breath.

God was a presence in that gauzy-white room, and my constant longing
	an eternity.
But Nicholas and Papa is one word, one name that lives on every day in
	each breath.

Nicholas Samaras, living in West Nyack, NY, is originally from Patmos, Greece, and writes from a place of permanent exile. His first book won the Yale Series of Younger Poets Award.

The Alzheimer's Man

Alan Steinberg

1
His daughter stands
at the door,
tasting the air.
All around, the leaves are burning,
bright flames of decay.
One day she will wander.
One day she will not come home.
She will find herself
another shelter.
In time he will say: This is good.
I have done what every father should.
In time he will see her children
lean from the door.
If he is lucky, he will go like this—
some quiet autumn morning,
smoke still on the leaves.
His going will be no more
than a first winter chill.

2
His father did not leave so.
He grew old and lost everything:
his eyes, his hair, his teeth, his reason.
It was he who stood by the door,
blindly gazing on the ruin
of another winter day—a city day filled
with wet and rancid snow.

3
He tells himself his father lacked
the grace to die as he should, in autumn,
with the sun burning the leaves.
On such a day, death passes
like a shadow across the sky,
a soul taking wing
like a bird flying south to prosper.
But he left him on a winter day,
the air thick, destitute, uneven,
with only a ragged sparrow given
to short and desultory flight.

4
So now this is how he would have it,
if we can have such things
as the season and the sorrow
of our passing.
It will be autumn.
There will be birds in the air.
His daughter will be standing
at the door gazing
at her own horizon.
Word will come of his leaving,
his rising up into the air
like a mist.
There will be nothing to say.
Nothing to regret.
There will be no silence to wall up.
The birds will be singing.

Alan Steinberg has published fiction (Cry of the Leopard, St. Martin's Press), poetry (Ebstein on Reflection, Idaho State Press), and drama (The Road to Corinth, Players Press). He teaches at SUNY Potsdam.

The Second Parlour

Anne Marie Todkill

Moira looked beautiful in her coffin. My mother couldn't get over it. She whispered to me, indecently, as we stood beside the casket, "She almost looks better than she did alive."

It was true enough. The normally dowdy Moira made a lovely corpse. Her skin was creamy and fine, like Irish porcelain. She lay in ruched white satin, her expression serene (this, too, was uncharacteristic), and she seemed almost angelic with her powdered cheeks and the delicate cloud of silver curls that framed her face.

Moira Lovell was the less congenial half of a childless couple who had lived next door to my parents ever since our little street of post-war bungalows was built. She spent her days indoors; every once in a while you would see her at the window, dressed in a shabby old caftan that suggested a determination to remain housebound and undisturbed in her one known activity, which was making crafts for Christmas bazaars. Most of these involved odd and unnecessary uses for crocheted granny squares, but odder by far was a sort of circular trivet made out of flattened cigarette packages cut and fitted together in a certain way. She showed me the knack of this once, to my mother's displeasure. "We're not having those filthy things on the table," my mother said, which made it impossible for me to mention that I liked the way the cardboard smelled and the interesting way the package designs worked out into parti-coloured pinwheels. If the original contents had filled Moira's lungs with soot, this impressed me less than the fact that she methodically changed brands throughout the year to keep up her colour schemes: Export A for green, du Maurier for red, Players for blue.

My mother had always felt rather cool toward Moira. She considered her to be, like the other women who "stayed at home" on our street, a potential liability, someone likely to shatter her peace with small talk or some request premised on an inability to drive or to sew or to endure solitude. My mother rarely sought company. The sharing of confidences was for girls, not married women. She was skeptical of friendship. She was certainly skeptical of the phone calls she occasionally received from next door: "Bea, why don't you ever come over for coffee? I'm so lonely." My mother would report this mockingly: "She's so l-l-o-h-h-h-nly. I don't have time to be lonely. Maybe if she thought about someone besides herself for a change she wouldn't feel so l-l-o-h-h-h-nly."

I doubt that I ever considered whether my mother was lonely, but it didn't escape me that her social life was more dutiful than joyful. In those years, when she was still well, my mother was the one who drove the ladies to the bowling league on Wednesday afternoon, who took another convoy to the hairdresser on Thursday, who hemmed skirts and took in waistbands, taking with as much annoyance as embarrassment the rolled-up two-dollar bills that Moira, among others, pressed into her hand. "I wish she wouldn't try to pay me," she would say. I can still hear the fretful intonation of Moira's voice as she stood in her dress shoes before the long mirror in my parents' bedroom, examining the effect of a new outfit. My mother would sit on the carpet, clenching a little row of straight pins between her lips as she tacked up Moira's hem against her tailor's ruler, a neat little contraption that stood vertical on the floor. "What do you think, Bea? Is it still a little long?"

"Turn," my mother would mutter through the pins. "OK, turn again. OK, now look."

"Oh Bea, you're right. That's fine there. You're so clever, Bea. Oh, Bea, how would I manage without you?"

Which must have irked my mother to no end. She had no tolerance for helplessness, unless it occurred in its natural form, in babies, small children, and men.

The Lovells' last years were overseen by two nieces who drove up at intervals from Napanee to check on matters at the house, then to make arrangements at the nursing home, and then to bury first Bill, and then Moira. When Moira was still living independently, The Nieces would phone occasionally to ask if all seemed well next door and to urge my parents to let them know if they had the slightest concern. Sometimes Moira would ring my mother up, asking if she would take her to the grocery store or pick up tea or eggs the next time she was out. Sometimes she would call for no reason other than to state how unwell she felt. At least this qualified as phoning for no reason as far as my mother was concerned. It used to shock me how scornful she was of those calls. I couldn't fathom why, after years of chauffeuring perfectly fit middle-aged women to bowling alleys and hair appointments and to Mass on First Fridays, she begrudged poor old Moira a lift to the grocery store. I was never sure what she disapproved of most. The self-disclosure? The self-pity? Or the way that Moira had brought sickness upon herself, with all those dirty cigarettes.

Whereas my mother's illness was just a bad draw. Although she was younger than Moira by eight or ten years, by that time her disease of the kidneys was well advanced. She now knew the reason for years of hypertension and fatigue, and she knew where her illness would take her. I used to think of her polycystic kidneys as blistered with retained emotion, leaking a little poison from time to time. I thought of my grandfather, many years dead, a man remembered for two things only: taciturn anger and a refusal to see doctors. I wondered how far faulty kidneys and a faulty temper had extended out from his inarticulate, undiagnosed history. I wondered if it reached as far as me.

It was not long after my mother entered the unbecoming phase of bitterness I struggle to describe that her kidneys failed her for good. She was reprieved for a time by dialysis. It was the beginning of a long ordeal, a chain of catastrophes that started with a bout of shingles that erupted in one eye and badly inflamed her face. An antiviral drug held the infection from her brain, or it nearly killed her, depending on whom you believed—the neurologist who had lost such a case to encephalitis, or the nephrologist who'd seen a patient poisoned like this before. Everything began with Z—zoster, Zovirax, zinc, and the name of the ophthalmologist. Z was a condemnatory letter: the end of the alphabet, the end of the road; the weight of that letter sank my mother into a coma; she was snagged on its sharp angles, caught in an algorithm of hazard that, afterward, I could never make her understand. But one bit of information did impress her: "In the middle of all this you may have had a couple of small strokes," the neurologist explained. "Or they might be old strokes on the scan. Mild strokes. It can happen without you being aware."

When The Nieces spotted us retreating from Moira's coffin they swept up effusively, hands extended. "Isn't Stan with you?" they asked, looking around for my father in a half-alarmed way, as if they were expecting bad news to pop out at them from nowhere.

"Oh, he's here," my mother said, nodding toward a clutch of people near the door. "I must say this is quite a turnout. When you get to be my age you wonder who'll be left to come to your funeral."

"You were such good neighbours to Moira and Bill," one of The Nieces said. "It was a comfort to us." I observed my mother's face closely. I think I was expecting her to wince. And so her response took me by surprise.

"Well, I'll be following Moira soon," she announced, throwing her voice a little, turning her gaze down the long double parlour to where our neighbour lay. "I won't be long behind her." I had the impression that several heads turned in our direction.

"Oh, no!" The Nieces exclaimed in a disbelieving tone that, to their credit, seemed entirely unfeigned. Against the evidence of my mother's sallow face and shrunken frame they blurted out their kindness: "You mustn't talk like that!"

"I'm on hemodialysis," she gravely informed them, as if this were the disease rather than an answer to it.

"Is that right?" the Nieces gasped. They steered my mother urgently to the nearest sofa and begged her to sit down.

And that was how my mother stole Moira Lovell's wake. A small twist in a small event, it was nonetheless stunning to me. Never in my life had I seen my mother make a bid for sympathy. Never had I seen her dramatize her situation. It was astonishing to see her in this light, queenly, crumpled, leaning against the armrest of a velvet sofa, recounting the history of her diagnosis, the progressive kidney failure, the two surgeries, one failed, both difficult, to create access in her arm, the hours she spent, three times a week, having her blood laundered, the appalling episode of shingles, her descent into near-death. She told her story to The Nieces as if it were a disclosure long hidden; as if her suffering had been entirely overlooked; as if her stoicism was a product not of her own strength but of the indifference of others.

I observed this performance from the proscenium doorway between the parlours, midway between The Nieces and Moira's coffin. My father sidled over to where I stood.

"What's your mother up to?"

"She's giving them the blow by blow."

"Oh my."

We stood transfixed by the emotive grouping on the couch.

"Of course," my father finally said, "one of The Nieces is a nurse. She might be interested."

Seeing my own embarrassment mirrored in my father, it was easier for me to judge it wrong.

"After all she's been through," I hissed, "I think she's entitled to a little attention."

Again the question presented itself. Who were my mother's confidantes? Who ever heard her story? No one. Until now, out of the blue, The Nieces.

In addition to sadness, in addition to remorse, I felt a sense of thwarted possession, as infantile as it was fierce.

There was my mother, dying without me.

I had no idea that sorrow could be so indignant.

A FEW YEARS after my mother died, when my daughter was a toddler, I had a bout of stomach flu. My daughter could not bear the sight of me lying down, immobile, inert, ignoring her. She railed against me, screaming Mommy as she pronounced it then, "Waabee, Waabee, Waabee," and beat her little fists on my stomach. Rolling on a wave of nausea, I turned my back to her, and she became all the more enraged. She flailed at my back, my shoulders, my head, and I was powerless to stop her frenzy. After a while she sat in a heap beside the bed, threw back her head, and howled like a little dog.

I recognized that howl. It was the sound I had heard rising within me on the day of Moira's wake. But to let such a wail of love escape my mouth would have been too strange, too startling, too childish, at the funeral of a woman I barely knew.

Anne Marie Todkill is an Ottawa-based writer and editor. Her publications include stories (Ars Medica), *poems* (Arc, The Malahat Review, Ars Medica), *and reviews* (LRC, Women's Review of Books). *She is a founding editor of* Open Medicine.

The Wong-Baker Scale

Gina P. Vozenilek

Tommy stands in our room, just past midnight. I can always hear the feet coming just before the lips place the "Mommy?" into the somnolent dark. I don't know how this should be so, since I can sleep right through a Saturday morning parade of children hurrying down to their cartoons and Cheerios. But, somehow, when they need me in the night, I hear easily. John, sleeping closer to the door, hardly notices that Tommy and I begin talking over the top of his turned shoulder.

"My ear hurts," says the boy in a thin voice. He speaks plainly, without whining, which always adds legitimacy to a midnight grievance.

I tell him I'm sorry to hear it, even though it means I was right. For weeks, all four kids have been passing around their germs like cards at a poker game; I am weary of the barking coughs and drippy noses and measured, sticky shots of Tylenol. When we tucked the boys in tonight, Tommy had felt warm to me. But his father had waved off my concern, and I'd grasped onto that more optimistic view of things.

Now here Tommy is, proof in Batman pajamas that I should have listened to my intuition. Mothers just know things about their children. Medical researchers have actually studied the effectiveness of a mother's touch for detecting a fever. They accurately make the call better than eight times out of ten merely by laying their hands on their child. My opinion should, therefore, trump John's, despite all his medical training.

But it proves hard to wake him, to solicit any opinion at all. He is drawing slow, loud breaths, trying to hang onto his sleep. I nudge him with my toe under the covers, irked.

"John. Tommy says his ear hurts. John?" Second toe poke.

"Whazza matta, buddy?" John slurs in exhalation, still not moving. Our bed is a high iron fortress, eclipsing Tommy from my sight. I imagine him standing there, alone below us on the cold wood floor, chilled by fever, waiting patiently for our arms to reach out and minister to him—touch his face, enfold his little body.

"My ear hurts, Daddy," he tries again.

"Oh. I'm sorry, buddy." And then to me, "Give'm some Motrin."

<u>What am I? The nurse?</u> The answer, of course, is always yes. I am the one who doles out the icepacks and the medicines and holds the heads as they throw up. I wash the soiled sheets and add the extra pillows and blankets, bring buckets and Kleenex and glasses of water and take them away again. I am the wiper of noses and the whisperer of solace and the bringer of comfort. <u>I am the mother</u>.

I swing my leaden feet over the edge of the bed and slide down to the floor, padding around to where Tommy waits. I administer a hug, feel his warm forehead again, and usher him to the bathroom. The passel of medicines still stands on the counter in its white plastic bin from a few nights ago. I find the right bottle and pour out two teaspoons of pink syrup, squinting at the tiny lines and numbers on the plastic cup. Then we plod back to his room, where I arrange blankets around Tommy and kiss his forehead.

"You'll feel better soon." I promise. "I hope you sleep well." I really do, because we all need the rest.

My sheets are just regaining their warmth when I hear Tommy coming again.

"<u>Daddy</u>? I can't sleep. My ear hurts too much." His voice is more plaintive now. The children are beginning to realize the differences between our parental authorities. The <u>nurse is soft and nice</u>, but the doctor has the solutions you really need. I don't disagree, but I often consider how that authority might be assigned in a house without a doctor-parent. If I had married a lawyer or a carpet salesman, I would be Nurse Nightingale *and* Doctor Spock. I was a pre-med, after all, before I got sidetracked into British literature and then came back full circle to Dr. Seuss.

"John?"

Grunt.

"John. Do you think you should look into his ear?"

Silence. The boy standing there.

Tommy's patience points up our slowness. I should get up again, but my head is so heavy on my pillow. Why isn't John moving yet? I want the doctor to do his stuff.

"John. Your son is standing right in front of you. His ear really hurts."

Now John sits up. I feel his resentment like a cold draft. We've talked about how worked up I get when one of the children falls ill. How I should relax and let him do his job. It's a matter of perspective. A sore throat chart in the emergency room hardly gets two minutes of his time. It isn't, I know, that John is indifferent to Tommy's pain. It's just that he has seen more and uglier faces of pain than I have. At the hospital he carries a little card in his pocket that depicts the faces of pain. It was designed to help patients rate their own degree of wretchedness. Shaped like a bookmark, it shows six line-drawings of faces representing the range from <u>no hurt to hurts worst</u>; in other words, a mini cartoon of the pain spectrum starting at *just fine, really,* and maxing out just before the brain bows into unconsciousness with *excruciating misery*. Patients—children and adults alike—are supposed to point to the face that best expresses how they feel. Doctors all over the world use this little tool called the <u>Wong-Baker Scale</u>. It helps bridge the essential gap that yawns between pain's reality and our ability to translate that pain meaningfully.

Of all the complaints registered in our house, we've been blessed never to get past the middle Wong-Baker grimace. Our eldest daughter, who needed an emergency appendectomy, went to the hospital with surprising stoicism. Mary observed the nurse unflinchingly as she inserted the IV into her pale arm and capped her with a blue paper puff on the way up to the surgical suite. Her first few post-op hours were hard, admittedly. "Dad!" she seethed. "You said the operation would make my tummy feel better, but it feels a lot worse!" Within a few hours, though, she forgave her father and dove into plenty of ice cream and video games. She came home two days later with a petite scar on her tummy and celebrity status in the first grade, like Ludwig Bemelmans's Madeline.

I ask again, "Are you going to look into that ear?" This annoys him even more than when I lead a waltz, but, as on a dance floor, I can't seem to keep my feet off his toes. He shuffles.

"Babe, there is no point to it. I am *not* going out of the house at this hour," John snaps.

"But tomorrow is the last day of vacation," I press. "Wouldn't it be good to give him the extra eight hours with antibiotics onboard? He'll feel that much better and might be ready for school."

I magnify my children's periodic discomforts by my inability to compare them to real hurt. John, by contrast, sees death and disease for a living, the weeping last face on the plastic bookmark. They come to him for help: sufferers of the varied and complicated kinds of pain that result from car wrecks, festering sores, end-stage cancer, gunshot wounds, knife fights, cardiac arrests, child abuse, and unsuccessful suicides—all manner of horrible hurt I am fortunate to be unable to describe. They overshadow any of the mundane maladies that come, like rainy days, to our house. And yet, *Who hurts worse?* is neither a question anyone can ever answer with certainty, nor is it a macabre contest to be won. "Pain," writes Victor Hugo, "is as diverse as man. One suffers as one can."

John, now sitting, is all shoulders in the dark. He hoists Tommy up in front of him and holds him fast. His head hangs down over his son, who is hidden from my view again. The two breathe together quietly. I cannot tell if John is assessing the patient or merely pressing the boy to his warm chest.

"Go on to your mother, Tommy," he says, his grogginess receding and his voice regaining its clear consonants. Tommy moves toward my pillow sleepily. John leaves us. A parallelogram of light slants onto the floor from the bathroom. He returns with his otoscope, its black conical beak pointing a pinprick of gold into the darkness. It aims into the ear and illuminates it red.

"Now you stay with Mommy. Don't fall asleep till I get back." He steps into his pants that are waiting like a fireman's on the floor and suits up. He is off to the pharmacy now for a prescription because I have guilted that otoscope into Tommy's ear. Now the infection is official; while it had been speculative, it could be treated with pain medicine and dealt with in the morning. The patient would really be no worse for it, and everyone could stay in warm beds till dawn. But now it is just bad form to make the little boy wait, the son so warm in his arms.

Outside it is raining when it really should be snowing. It is the kind of night when the air swims with a dampness that clings and burrows with you into your coat. I can hear the rain falling onto the slope of the roof now. A few nights earlier I was startled by the thunderous scraping sound of the first puzzle-piece of ice melting loose and sliding off the shingles over my head. John was working the night shift then, and I was alone in the high bed. Now I am snuggling Tommy closer and devising a strategy to keep us both awake as promised. I feel bad for John out in the middle of night in the cold rain; the least I can do is deprive myself of sleep in solidarity.

"How about we read a book?" I ask, clicking on the bedside lamp.

Tommy brightens. "An *I Spy*," he decides. He retrieves the book he wants and we begin reading. Just like the old road-trip game to pass the time, an *I Spy* book is about perceiving hidden things and solving little riddles. It is colourful distraction. I raise Tommy up on the pillows and we put our heads together.

As we look at the page in the small circle of light, I can feel Tommy's discomfort by the way he fidgets and squirms in the crook of my arm. Sometimes he turns away from the page and lays his pink cheek against my chest. "When will Daddy be back?"

"Soon, honey."

He is small next to me, the sweetest fraction of his father. We could curl up and drift off and enter the same dream. Tommy and I share a drowsy contentment: one needing comfort and one giving it, both grateful for the other being there at this late moment under the covers. The needing and the needed. In this earache night, our son wants simple things from his father and me. And we have them to give, each in our own way. I know someday there will be different kinds of hurts that neither of us will be able to fix so easily. In a flush of something between selfishness and gratitude, I am glad for this night. "Look! *There's* the third red sword," I rally. "Can you find the ostrich?"

Time passes slowly. Just as we begin to grow too tired for the crowded images before our eyes, we hear the key in the door downstairs. Tommy scrambles out of bed and down the stairs to meet his father. I expect the oak steps to creak again momentarily under sleepy footsteps as the pair drag back up towards bed. I wait. No creak comes. Instead, I hear a rustling of bags. At first it is the paper tear of the prescription envelope, but that is followed by the rustling of plastic bags. Still no feet on the stairs. I head downstairs to investigate.

Tommy sits on a stool at the kitchen counter, drinking chocolate milk straight from a quart container bought especially for him. He is colouring a picture with his dad in a fresh sketch pad. A splintered rainbow of finely sharpened colored pencils spills from a new zippered case onto the butcher block.

"What do we have here?" I ask quietly, surveying the curious collection of new goodies around the bright kitchen. I am careful to modulate my voice, to cover my surprise at this spontaneous late night art party. The clock above says 1:45 a.m. Of course, we should all be asleep now. But I know without being told that there is special medicine in this kitchen, beyond the chalky pink pills in the tube. I know it is important to follow John's lead now.

"I took care of some things," John replies with a shrug, looking up at me.

We bend silently towards each other. Tommy sits between us. He scribbles a grey sky with a pointy sun shining through the corner. John works out a fine bear. It might be coming out of hibernation. Tommy grounds the scene with a swath of sideways grass and begins an oval. A turtle emerges with a purple shell. I add a tree with arching branches, which Tommy covers for me with a hazy green canopy.

"Put some birds in it," he says. I do my best blue birds, tiny beaks upraised in song, or perhaps for a worm. We work like that quietly, filling the page together. On the clock that hangs above our heads, two hands silently sweep away the time.

Gina Pribaz Vozenilek is a freelance science writer and managing editor of Sport Literate *Magazine (www.sportliterate.org). Her essays have appeared there, in* Notre Dame Magazine, *and* Brain, Child. *She lives and writes in Park Ridge, IL.*

Denial

Gina Wilch and Ruby Roy

Gina's Story

Most parents start with success: "Congratulations, you have a beautiful, healthy baby." We started with "Your son has bacterial meningitis. He's had strokes and most likely will not live."

There is a delicate balance between hope and skepticism. After absorbing all the facts, I too had a very hard time believing he would ever be "normal." My husband and I learned very early just how essential hope and belief are. We would only be failing our son—and our son would fail—if *we* couldn't believe in him.

Dr. Roy started out as just our pediatrician. Nine years ago we *saw* her skepticism, respectfully backed up by the facts. She then became our success marker, as someone who saw Justin every so often and reflected his growth back to us. Then, when she told me about her son, I realized she and I were not so different after all.

Justin has to go about learning most things a different way. There are some things his disabilities prevent him from doing very well, but we always tried. Riding a bike was difficult, but singing, playing the piano, and the computer are strong abilities. I know some very "normal" people who can't do that. If you spend too much time focusing on what he may *still* never do, you will miss today. We appreciate what most parents may take for granted.

Most people look at denial as a negative word. Denial is what made it possible for Justin to come running around the corner in our kitchen carrying a book that he opened to read to me. That entire sentence, broken apart, embodies the perseverance of every one of his therapists, teachers, and doctors, their hope, and, yes, their denial. "Maybe this one child will make it." Denial is often our drive. It is our silent protector.

It is the small triumphs that count. The other day we were in line and Justin, who is visually impaired, read every word on the sign in front of him. The parent behind me did not notice the lump in my throat or the catch in my voice when I said, "Good job, pal," knowing that it took nine years of blood, sweat, and tears to reach the point where he could read that sign. I was "in the moment."

I came across a quote shortly after he was born. I am not sure who wrote it, but it echoes in my head almost daily. "That which you believe becomes your world." Because I denied, I believed, and that belief became Justin's world.

Ruby's Story

Denial is not a river in Egypt. That's a medical joke—used to denigrate a patient who refuses to "face reality." Reality, in this case, is our medical point of view, which is usually grim. Doctors do not want to be accused of giving false hope—we can't be sued if the patients are already expecting the worst. We dole out hope carefully, in statistics.

This is ironic, because another medical joke is that there are three kinds of lies: lies, damn lies, and statistics. (We keep that joke to ourselves, a medical secret.) To our patients, statistics are presented as Truth, as Scientific Fact, worthy of Belief. "You have a 70 per cent five-year survival." "The operation has a 95 per cent success rate." "There's a less than 10 per cent complication rate." "Your chance of having a child with a heart problem if you are healthy is only 1 per cent." "Your chance of having a second child with a heart condition is only 2 per cent." Not much difference between 1 per cent and 2 per cent, is there? But what if I told you that your chance of having a second affected child is double that of the first? And if you already have a child with a heart problem, your "1 per cent risk" has already happened. When medicine becomes playing the odds, it ceases to be a hopeful way of living your life.

I learned about the positive uses of denial from one of my clinic families. Justin was born at a small community hospital at full term and was discovered to have bacterial meningitis two days later. The hospital should have suspected this at birth, but chose not to do the spinal tap, because he looked fine initially. By the time he was transferred to our academic facility, he most certainly looked far from fine. The infection had attacked his brain, and he had had multiple seizures and breathing problems and was in a coma. After three weeks of maximal intensive care, the parents—Gina and Don—were told that the time had come to give up. They were going to take baby Justin off the ventilator and they expected him to be dead within twelve hours. One month later, Gina and Don brought this baby to me for his two-month check up. They were, as I assessed, after looking through the hospital notes and the brain scans, completely in denial. They felt that Justin was a "miracle child" and were committed to believing that he would be normal. I had enough empathy for what they had been through to know that they would not trust any prognosis for Justin's future that I gave, after the ICU doctors had been so wrong, so I consciously refused to make any predictions. His scans indicated that Justin would be blind and vegetative—certainly not that he would have any kind of meaningful quality of life. But Gina refused to believe this and brought to each visit a chronicle of what Justin had learned to do. She believed that he could see her, and that he was smiling responsively. Our ophthalmologist was skeptical, and so was I. Gina started him in treatments to strengthen his muscles and aid his development and became a therapist for him. Whatever the professionals did in their hourly sessions, she continued, so that this child was getting therapeutic stimulation for twelve to sixteen hours of every day. And he made progress. She was tireless and unfailingly hopeful. The time and energy she devoted to her son was incredible. I was impressed, but more by her as a mother than by him as a child. As I applauded his progress and supported her role, my skeptical medical voice was telling me, "He may be able to do this, but he'll never be normal."

At Justin's four-year physical visit I saw him for the first time as he really was. I walked through the door into the exam room and sat on the chair and Justin walked over, climbed onto my lap, took my stethoscope from around my neck and said, not clearly, but unmistakably, "Hi, Doctor Roy!" I finally saw a child with some physical and speech delays, with some vision problems, but clearly an active, personable, and charming little boy. Not a vegetable. I had been in denial myself. He had improved miraculously—and was not at all in the dismal state that his lab tests and brain scans had predicted. I had not been alone in my skepticism. Perhaps, since miracles aren't something doctors can take credit for, they are hard for us to see, even when they are happening right under our noses.

And so I've learned from this family that there is an upside to denial—to living in a place that does not succumb to medical reality. Denial has allowed me to raise my own son for eleven years to feel like a normal kid, unrestricted by the limitations of the diagnosis of Ebstein's anomaly. It's allowed him the freedom to play soccer, to earn a purple belt in tae kwon do, to bike eight miles along a trail, without my wondering if his tiredness is due to his heart, or fearing that every twinge is a cardiac arrhythmia. Denial serves as an antidote to hypochondriasis. It's not lying—my son has been aware of his heart-valve problem since he was five years old. But it's about not dwelling on it and its ramifications every day.

I have come out of denial for two days of every year since my son was a baby—those two days are the day prior to his yearly cardiology appointment and the day of the appointment itself. And for those two days, I live in fear. I think about his risks of heart failure, of stroke, or of sudden death. I worry about the degree of heart enlargement that they will see on cardiac ultrasound, or if they will pick up an arrhythmia on EKG. I worry about risks of medicine and of surgery, neither of which will cure him. And there is a part of this fear that is irrational, but one all parents would understand—that something is wrong with my child and I am powerless to help him, to fix it, that I have failed as a mother, the one who bore him and yet could not prevent this congenital problem. Countless doctors have asked me about drug use during my pregnancy—trying to find a cause, something or someone to blame. Despite not using drugs or alcohol in pregnancy, I, as the mother, am responsible. "Reality" is the emotional hell of fear, hypochondria, blame, and guilt. Myself, I'd rather live in Egypt.

Ruby Roy is an academic pediatrician who specializes in the care of special needs children at Loyola University Medical Center in Chicago. Her son with Ebstein's anomaly is doing well after recent cardiac surgery.

Gina Wilch lives in Elk Grove Village, Illinois, with her husband Don and two kids, Justin and Sarah. She serves on panels for both the educational and medical needs of special needs kids.

Part 3: Practitioners

Introduction

> We have art so that we do not perish by the truth.
> –Nietzsche

Physicians and other healthcare practitioners are trained in how to approach the body with knowledge. A clinical framework is imparted through training, to capture the body with its analytic, scientific and technical terms, in order to pin this medicalized body down and subject it to the scrutiny that one hopes will lead to "truth" in the form of the correct diagnosis and treatment. Terms and words like incisive, probing, procedure, evidence, examination, lay bare this process of reducing and fragmenting in order to know and to treat. And yet, in the close space of the clinical encounter physicians, nurses and other practitioners are confronted by the body in all of its fleshiness, fragility, states of decay and complex humanity. In these instances when one is called to lay hands on the flesh of another, the gap between knowledge and truth can be sometimes astounding, sometimes joyful and sometimes bewildering.

The clinician-writers of the stories and narratives in this section take us into the space of the clinical encounter, spaces as diverse as an emergency department, a hospital room, a freighter filled with refugees, a room at a dying man's home, and a decaying general ward at a hospital. We are given a vantage from the clinician's position-takings, following the physician on rounds, or shadowing the wandering of an anaesthetist taking night call at a hospital, or looking at the patient and body through the lens of a camera. Most provocatively, however, we are given a glimpse into what happens when medical knowledge meets the fleshy truth of the body, when the subjectivity of the encounter with the patient-as-person overflows the template of scientific knowledge. In such moments, we can look away, can hold up knowledge as a shield, employing medical jargon like the physician is tempted to do in "The Texture of a Word," as Dr Jack Diggs in "Accident Room" acknowledges, "treating the disease [is] easier than treating the person." Similarly, we can, as Paul Whang confesses, "depersonalize" the situation and become "coldly clinical," a "medical bureaucrat."

Instead of this refusal, this barrier against the other, however, each of these narratives represents an attempt to bridge the gap between the objectivity of clinical practice and the subjectivity of encountering another in their most fragile and most open state – to approach the other rather than distance oneself. The space of the narrative allows the clinician to be with the other, and to tolerate this, even when the limitations of their knowledge are exposed, and when there is no medical intervention that will "cure." Many of the narratives are also about being with one's self as a clinician, grappling with the weight of one's medical decisions, and living with one's mistakes. This encounter with the humanity of others, and with one's own humanity, is a "truth" beyond medical knowledge, and these narratives help us not only to survive these truths of the body and of mortality, as Nietzsche suggests, but to survive them together.

Allison Crawford, MD

Accident Room

Jay Baruch

Late Friday afternoon, Doc Owens phones Dr. Jack Diggs in the Pickton Hospital Emergency Department. "I'm sending a patient to your accident room, young Jack. Name is Brick Rolfson. You should know a few details before he shows up."

"Go ahead, Doc," Jack says, sounding cheerful and eager, though his spine stiffens as if bracing for a blow.

The demented, the hypochondriacs, the crazies all belong to Doc Owens. Most live in nursing facilities and group homes, the cluster of square grey high-rises overlooking the winding and slow-moving Pickton River and the red brick power plant that feeds it. Loneliness and constipation, Doc Owens believes, sit at the root of most of their complaints—from muscle pains to headaches to insomnia. If reassurance and laxatives can't improve their symptoms, he sends them to the "accident room," where the real source of the problem is often identified—a pneumonia, a bladder infection, side effects from all the medications he keeps adding on, more being better.

Accident room? An antiquated term for the Emergency Department, in this country anyway, and Jack knows he needs to set Doc straight. But he just finished his residency. He's new to Pickton. How can he make that point without insinuating that the elder clinician's skills are dated as well? So Jack squeezes the pen into the pill-shaped notepad and obediently follows Doc's story.

Brick fell from his recliner yesterday evening. This morning, Sylvie calls Doc's office, insisting her husband get looked at. He's lumbering about their second floor apartment above "Brick's Place," mentioning his lower back.

"Mentioning?" asks Jack, but Doc's story takes a detour on Brick's Place. "Every year it's voted Best Pub and Best Burger by *Night Out Pickton*," Doc says with great pride. "You should take the wife. You can't consider yourself a local until you've eaten there a thousand times." Jack listens and waits. He can't find a neat place in the conversation to politely reroute Doc back to the problem at hand. "Did you know that Brick's left arm once hurled major league lightning?" Doc recounts warmly. "Brick made it to AAA with the Sox before being drafted into Vietnam." "Is that so?" says Jack, by now wanting to thrust his skinny arm through the phone line and shake the starch from Doc's shirt collar. But Jack no longer works at "The Pit," the hectic and combative inner city ER where he trained. When Jack and his wife first visited Pickton Hospital two months earlier, their eyes widened as they ascended the dreamy, serpentine drive lined with landscape roses and wood chips. Even the blaring red "Emergency" sign was softened by a train of English ivy. The Pickton Medical Society welcomed Jack with a luncheon, where Doc Owens, the former chief of the hospital staff, gave him a slap on the back, a wink, and a bottle of Bordeaux, a gift that he held clumsily in his hands, like the Titleist golf clubs his wife gave him for Christmas two years earlier. She hoped he'd learn to play. He needed a hobby. Now, the golf clubs and unopened wine—gentle reminders of the expectations of others—furnish a dark corner in an otherwise spare panelled basement.

The nurse in charge of the ER nudges Jack to hang up and get moving. Patients are backing up. Jack clears his throat, a startling phlegm-dredging scrape. Doc pauses. "Excuse me," says Jack. "Did Brick pass out? Does his neck hurt?"

"No, not at all. I don't think so," Doc says, uncertain yet firm. "I added a stool softener a few days ago. Maybe that has something to do with it."

Jack scribbles the words *fall* and *soft stools*. The words dare him to make sense of them. To Jack, they reveal more about Doc's loose mind than Brick's physical condition. He thinks about Doc's oil portrait hanging in a basement corridor alongside other hospital notables, his snowy white hair, watery blue eyes, and warm smile perched between the rehabilitation unit and the staff cafeteria. He wonders what utility remains in people once they live long enough to be preserved on canvas.

"Any other problems?" he asks, hoping to bring the conversation to a close.

"I told you about his lungs," Doc says. "Tumours like golf balls. Inoperable."

"No! You didn't." Jack scratches his forehead. "Is he DNR?"

Doc Owens chuckles into the phone. "Why do you always ask about do-not-resuscitate orders? Don't you want to save anyone?"

"Not if the patient is terminal and wants to die quietly."

"Check the back, Jack," says Doc, dismissively, as if scolding a child. "Get an X-ray. Make the wife happy." His voice trails away. He tells someone in his office to "hold on to your trousers, I'll be there in a few shakes."

"Brick overdid it," Doc Owens tells Jack. "He still works the bar every night. Believes Sylvie needs the help. But that woman doesn't need any help from anyone."

BRICK ROLFSON'S WIFE immediately corrects Doc Owens when they arrive in the Emergency Department. "He didn't fall off his chair," she snaps, her red lipstick too bold. "He collapsed getting into it." She leans forward beside Brick's gurney, adjusts the braided silver ponytail that drops down to her boyish hips. "My husband was blown off a bridge in Vietnam, sent home, and he re-enlisted. If the chair wasn't booby-trapped, he didn't fall off."

She pokes the air to punctuate each point. The sleeveless blouse tucked into a matching beige skirt reveals wiry, muscular arms. "And my name is Sylvia, not Sylvie."

"I'm sorry, ma'am," says Jack.

"I'm not a ma'am." Even with fluffy bedroom slippers she appears lean and ferocious. "Are you a doctor? You look twelve."

"Easy, Mom," says Candice, sitting cross-legged next to her mother, reading a paperback with a blurry cover. Candice is heavy, with round cheeks, and green eyes that sparkle with kindness. Or so Jack hopes. He recognizes her from Johnson's Bakery. Squeezed into the white apron, she serves up fresh breads, pastries, and lottery tickets. The tinselled shop window flanks Bruno's Cards and Things, where Mylar balloons float in the front window and XXX movies and snap-on dildos pack the back aisles. Bruno's is the only store in town that carries the *New York Times*. Jack stops by almost every morning, still tethered to what he seeks to escape.

"He was watching the ball game," Candice says. "Suddenly he stood up, stared at the television, and somehow lost his balance sitting down." She slices a Polaroid of two infants into the book to mark her spot. "He mentioned his back." Candice stares at her father with a worried expression that pleads with him to elaborate.

"What do you mean 'mentioned?'" Jack asks.

"My husband never complains," Sylvia interrupts, her voice heating up. "If he mentions something, it's bad."

Jack nods, draws a deep breath, and studies Brick lying on the stretcher, apparently content to let the conversation snake around him. He has a sledgehammer head, fleshy jowls, a bulbous nose threaded with veins. A bartender's face, Jack thinks, beaten and trustworthy. This face would lead you into inebriation and make certain a cab or friend returns you safely home.

"May I take a look at your back?" Jack asks Brick.

"Forget the back," says Brick. "Nothing's wrong with the back."

"Why did you mention it?" Jack asks, flicking a look at Sylvia, his intolerance for them primed because they belong to Doc Owens. He pauses. "What is bothering you?"

"Nothing." Brick tightens his jaw, lowers his head. He pulls away when Candice grabs his hand and tries to bring his hairy knuckles to her lips. Sylvia sits stone-faced, nodding at her slippers. Jack waits. "Talk to each other. Maybe you don't need to be here," says Jack, "I'll step out," and leaves the exam room.

He scrubs his hands vigorously at a nearby sink. Sylvia approaches.

"He hardly eats," she says, surprising Jack with her tone. Did she blame him for Brick's twenty-pound weight loss?

"There are special shakes you can buy. Doc Owens can help you with that."

Smacking his wet hands with a paper towel, Jack startles when Sylvia throws her hands into the air. "That's what Doc Owens did when I asked if the tumour had anything to do with his appetite. He changed the subject, zeroed in on his bowels. His bowels! You can set your watch to his colon. Now I ask you, and you toss me back to Doc Owens. What is this, a game of hot potato?"

"That's not fair," says Jack, about to say something rude he might regret later, when she kindly steps aside to allow a nurse to pass. She returns to the same spot, under the same fluorescent light, with the same incendiary glow to her cheeks. But now her rage has dissipated enough to allow Jack to see the desperation hiding underneath.

"What's going on with my husband?" asks Sylvia, shielding her eyes, as if wary of the information she desires.

"He fell. Doc wants me to check him out."

"That's not what I mean." She holds him in her grey, unblinking eyes.

"Brick is ill." Jack's mouth is dry. Was the truth his to spend? "He's very ill."

"You're wrong," says Sylvia.

"Inoperable lung cancer."

"No! A tumour, not cancer."

Jack's jaw falls slack. "Is that what Doc said, or what you heard?"

The corner of Sylvia's mouth twitches. "How do you know all this?"

"Doc told me."

"Why didn't he tell us? He said the X-ray showed walking pneumonia. The tumour was a 'by-the-way.' We shouldn't worry. He'd watch it. Watch it?"

Jack feels challenged to respond, to enlarge and justify her smouldering bitterness. He raises his eyebrows, invites her to continue, but it's clear his silence disappoints her. "You're twelve, you probably don't remember Dr. Riggins. When he died suddenly, we became Doc's hand-me-downs." She swallows hard. "The wrong doctor had the stroke."

"Doc Owens is a good man," says Jack.

"House scotch," she scoffs.

"What?" Jack asks, aware he's revealing that he's not much of a drinker, and this fact most likely will diminish him further in Sylvia's eyes.

Sylvia shakes her head. "Well, scotch. Cheap stuff, but it's better than nothing."

Jack bites his tongue, fights the urge to agree with her. Pain replaces words; pain he can tolerate. When the pain subsides, he excuses himself, steps outside into the ambulance bay. The sobering night breeze carries cigarette smoke and skunk from the municipal golf course across the street. Workers under kleig lights are digging up the tenth hole. Rumour is that the town is expanding Pickton Cemetery. Everyone talks about it and no one believes it. It's a curious counter to the common knowledge that the size of Doc Owen's practice has exceeded his diminishing abilities. Yet this fact is considered only obliquely, acknowledged with knowing expressions, never words. Jack imagines how "The Eternal Back Nine" would play out and visualizes tombstone foursomes of Doc's former patients packing the fairways.

JACK CALLS Doc's office, expecting the service operator who will page him. Even though it's 7 p.m. on a Friday, Doc is busy seeing patients, clearly annoyed that Brick remains in the "accident room."

"I accidentally told the wife Brick was dying," Jack says curtly.

"She knows about the tumour," says Doc. "The guy smokes like a chimney. They know. I didn't have to tell them."

Jack cups his hand over the phone so he isn't overheard. "The ER isn't a warm and fuzzy place to have a discussion about death."

"My office isn't warm and fuzzy, either." Doc Owens hisses into the phone. "Jesus, Jack. Why are you yanking my yingyang over this?"

He doesn't answer right away. Through the open door he catches Sylvia wringing a washcloth, pressing it against her husband's forehead, which Brick promptly removes. Candice squeezes her father's hand, rests her face against their messy ball of interlocking fingers. Brick turns to his daughter with a wry grin, appreciating her gesture and acknowledging its uselessness. Jack begins thinking: Did Doc Owens really decide to ignore the tumour and let Brick die? Many of Doc's patients are dying, or believe they're dying. This inexorable fate might discourage most physicians, those preoccupied with curing their patients; but for physicians in the sunset of their careers, or those who were never clinically strong, dying patients offer protection, a measure of comfort. Along with the body, sealed in the casket and lowered six feet into the soil, was everything the physician didn't know or do.

"In my day, we didn't treat people to death," Doc says, breaking Jack's silence. "When your time came, that was it."

"YOU SHOULD STAY in the hospital," Jack tells Brick. "At least overnight."

"What's wrong?" asks Sylvia.

"For observation. We'll watch him, maybe run some tests," says Jack.

Sylvia points to the scuffed linoleum floor. "He'll be here?"

"We'll get him a bed upstairs."

"Doc Owens will still be his doctor?"

"Of course."

"No. Not 'of course.'"

Brick closes his eyes. "It doesn't matter."

"We want a different doctor," Sylvia says.

"It doesn't matter," says Brick, forcefully now.

"Couldn't you be his doctor?" asks Candice, trying to mediate.

Jack steps back, thinks of Doc doing rounds on his patients every morning by 5:45, the dandruffed collar of his suit pulled askew across his stooped shoulders by the stethoscope stuffed into the jacket pocket. Jack lowers his voice. "Doc is a decent man."

"House scotch," Sylvia lashes out.

Brick's eyes spring open, round and glassy.

"What is it, Dad?" Candice asks, dabbing sweat from his cheeks.

"It's nothing," says Brick.

"It's not nothing," says Sylvia. "Why won't you talk to me?"

Jack feels her looking his way. To whom is she directing that question?

THREE HOURS LATER, still waiting in the ER for a hospital bed to come available, Brick begins breathing quickly, his skin paler than before. Jack marches his stethoscope up and down Brick's sweaty back. He hears sounds like crumpling sheets of paper. He's disturbed by this new finding. Sylvia and Candice step away, holding hands.

"How do you feel?" Jack asks.

Brick gives Jack a thumbs-up.

"Why is he breathing so hard?" asks Sylvia.

"Pulmonary edema." Jack twists the stethoscope into his white coat.

Candice nods. Sylvia doesn't pretend to understand. "Say again?"

"His lungs are filling with fluid."

"Why is this happening?" asks Sylvia.

Jack nervously leafs through the chart. "I can't say."

"Why not?"

"I mean I don't know," Jack bites back. "I can't piece this whole thing together." He pinches his tired eyes. How can he admit how lost his is? Then a nurse slips an EKG into his hands and Jack, embarrassed, breaks into an honest smile. The normal heart speaks in rhythmic, lean geometry. Brick's tracings reveal mountainous slopes, the silent screams of an acute heart attack.

"What's so funny?" asks Sylvia. Jack knows a smile at such a critical moment is inappropriate and deserves an apology, but he's truly elated and can't hide it. "Let's start over," Jack tells Brick, confident in the way people are when they have insider information. "Are you having chest pain?"

Brick responds with the slow, barely perceptible waggle of his index finger he uses to cut off drunks who believe they can hold one more. Jack leans into Brick's ear, holds his breath against the metallic odour wafting from Brick's cracked mouth. "You should've mentioned your chest," he whispers.

A grin splits Brick's tightly sealed lips. Rather than sly, he appears embarrassed at being found out, and grateful. The lung cancer is a red herring, Jack thinks to himself, the back pain a ruse, a strategy to get to the hospital. This way, Sylvia or Candice or the grandchildren wouldn't have the shock of discovering his body sprawled across the apartment floor or rocking stiffly in his chair. As Jack watches Brick's bluish lips purse around each shallow breath, he wonders how long Brick has been enduring the chest pain, concealing it from his family.

"Do something," Sylvia cries. "Don't just stand there."

Brick freezes Jack with his dark eyes, wet and threatening, in which Jack sees the steely soldier, the once-promising baseball player, the stern bartender—a man savvy to codes of discretion. The EKG traces an ominous and probably fatal path. The heart attack was kept hidden for a reason.

"Let's talk about DNR," says Jack, guessing that Doc Owens never raised it, and that Brick, by his actions, has declared his readiness to die.

He explains chest compressions, a breathing tube in the windpipe, other life-sustaining treatment. "Do you want me to do these things if your heart or your lungs stop working?"

Brick shrugs his shoulders. Jack feels a cold chill. If Brick is intent on dying, why did he respond with a shrug, as if being asked whether he wants bar nuts or pretzels with his pint?

"Stop talking," says Sylvia to Jack. "Help him."

"I need to know your wishes, or I'll assume you want everything done." Jack presses Brick, tilting his head, trying to communicate without betraying their secret. Finally, he asks, "What do you want me to do, Brick?"

Brick rests his head back against the gurney like a first-class passenger just before liftoff. He's breathing with his entire body, as if sucking air through a flat straw, but he appears strangely comfortable. Jack is stymied. How could he be so sure of himself moments before? The diagnosis wasn't the answer, only the spark that set fire to the question, "Did Brick really want to die?"

"You're watching my husband die," says Sylvia, neck vessels thickening. "How can you do that?" She squirms when Candice tries to embrace her. "Just like Owens."

That's when Jack finally gives in. He pushes his hands into latex gloves, glances at Sylvia, and responds with a litany of drug orders. The nurse flies about Brick's body, syringes loaded. Brick's heart will soon stop, regardless of what is done. But Jack exhales. A deep calm warms his veins. Each step is automatic, treating the disease easier than treating the person, but he can't shake the shame that what he's doing is wrong.

Jack believes in the beauty of a good death. In Brick's case, it means oxygen and morphine, calming Brick's air hunger until his breathing finds a tranquil groove. He waits beside Sylvia and Candice until the heartbeat in Brick's bulky chest goes silent.

Maybe Sylvia turns to Jack. "I knew something wasn't right," she says. "Thank you."

Perhaps Jack squeezes her hand.

But none of this happens. There are chest compressions and a breathing tube sitting between his vocal cords preventing any last hope of Brick saying goodbye.

The thrill of rescue pulls him along and Jack can't escape it, nor does he want to. Brick's blood pressure drops. Jack reacts. He knows exactly what is called for. The drugs keep coming. Doc's laxatives will be equally ineffective, but Sylvia doesn't know that, nor does Candice. Jack's light-headed by this realization, nauseated too. He wonders if, and how, he'd ever be forgiven. Candice's wide face, thunderstruck, flushed with confidence and hope, answers him.

JACK CALLS Doc Owens. Wails echo in the background.

"What's that?" Jack asks, checking a wall clock—10:30 p.m.

"The Sirens of Mountain View."

"What?"

"Nursing home rounds."

"Brick Rolfson is dead," Jack says, deciding to come right out and tell him. "We coded him."

"It's for the best," Doc says dispassionately. "Brick was a fighter."

Jack chokes on that comment. "It's for the best?"

They share a tense silence. Jack needs to tell Doc exactly what happened, every detail. Brick didn't fight. Jack beat him up. He must confront Doc; never again will he dump a mess into his lap and expect him to clean it up. But it's late at night and Doc isn't home in bed. He's attending to his patients, probably doing the best job he can. And what would happen to these patients if Doc weren't there?

Jack quickly changes the subject. "Why call it Mountain View? This town is flat."

"Don't know, Jack. Why do they call it a nursing home? I've been rounding for an hour and haven't seen a single nurse."

Nervous silence fills the phone line. "Is Sylvie there?"

"She's with Brick. And her name is Sylvia."

"Say again?"

"Sylvia, not Sylvie."

"Right, right! Put her on, will you?" he asks.

Jack lowers the receiver and calls for her.

"Tell him to fuck off," she says.

Jack gets back on the phone. "She's pretty upset."

AFTERWARD, outside Brick's room while her daughter phones relatives, Sylvia surprises Jack by shaking his hand. "You did everything," she says, looking through him, as if he's obstructing her line of vision to the future. "Stop by Brick's Place, we'll take good care of you and your wife."

"Come by the bakery the next time you pick up your paper," Candice warmly offers.

"I'm sorry for your loss," Jack tells them, uneasy that they know of his wife and at least some of his routine. He avoids them as they wait for the funeral director to pick up the body. In his mind, he's giving them room to grieve. But he feels guilty, somehow at fault. Uncertainty shadows him as he dodges about the accident room seeing to other patients. It follows him home. He can't sleep. Perhaps that's really what the wine is for. He pads down the cool basement steps and stealthily feels his way without turning on the light.

Jay Baruch practises emergency medicine in Rhode Island and teaches medical ethics at Brown Medical School. His fiction has appeared or will in Another Toronto Quarterly, Other Voices, Inkwell, Fetishes, Issues Magazine, *and* Segue.

Tale of a T-shirt

Susan Croft

In October 2006, Brian Ouma arrived at Kisumu Airport in the western port city of Kisumu, Kenya, to greet Brenda Gallie. As he and Abby White stood watching the ponderous puddle-jumper trundle down the runway towards the terminal, he wondered how much they would achieve before Brenda's return to Canada a week later, and Abby's return to England in three weeks. All he knew was that their hopes were high and their plan, to raise awareness of how to recognize retinoblastoma in children while it was still treatable, was ambitious.

After a long, tedious, and futile search for her luggage, Brenda emerged into the arrivals lounge. Abby, her friend and colleague of just two years, introduced her to a tall man with an engaging smile, who carried a sandy-coloured T-shirt draped over one arm.

"Brenda Gallie, Brian Ouma," Abby introduced. "Brian's agreed to give us a hand with launching the project."

Returning Brian's smile, Brenda shook his hand. His grip was strong and sure, his smile genuine, and his greeting heart-felt. He and Abby were already wearing their T-shirts—replicas of the one he pushed into her hands. Aside from the fact that this was now her only change of clothes, she felt a rush of pleasure at seeing it. This, after all, was why she had come: to wear a T-shirt, make a statement, make a difference.

The difference, Abby thought, was that North Americans generally ignored each other's T-shirts, while Africans took T-shirt slogans to heart. Standing beside Brenda at the podium during their first presentation, she marvelled at the effectiveness of the idea. Why wouldn't it be effective, though? It had worked before, for malaria and AIDS, and it certainly seemed to be working again now for retinoblastoma. She looked out over the sea of faces. Abby couldn't see well: Her own retinoblastoma had destroyed much of her vision by the age of two years, and eventually one eye was removed when she was twenty-five. She knew though—Brenda had whispered it to her while they were being introduced in two different languages—that the forty T-shirts they had brought had already been handed out and there were still many people who wanted one. Next time they would have to bring more.

It wasn't just family members and doctors—people who encountered the childhood eye cancer—who filled the little rooms in which Brenda, Abby, and Brian gave their presentation. Nurses, family friends, and members of the general population attended as well. Everyone wanted to know about the white reflection in the pupil, like the gleam of a cat's eye, that was clearly visible in the eye of the child that fronted the T-shirt. This strange phenomenon was called leukocoria and was caused by the flash of a camera or other bright light reflecting off the tumour that grew unnoticed at the back of an infant's eye. This white glow was often the first indication to a parent that something was wrong. In Canada and England, simple tests and reliable treatments could be used to save a child. Here though, in Kisumu, Kenya, options were limited and the death rate among affected children was 90 per cent, compared to 4 per cent in developed countries.

Another hot room. Brenda shifted uncomfortably as she spoke, pausing every now and again to let the two translators catch up. The heat didn't bother Abby. Kenya was her spiritual home. Her father had been born here, had been diagnosed here in 1946 before being transported to England for treatment—removal of both eyes and radiotherapy. Time and time again he had told her how lucky he was to have the option of receiving medical care in the United Kingdom. If he had been an African child, like Rati, he probably wouldn't have survived.

Rati hadn't survived. That beautiful little girl had been diagnosed too late and without enough knowledge in her home country of Botswana. When Abby heard her story, she pulled every string she could to get her to Brenda in Toronto. They had been too late. Treatment in Canada gave Rati a year of high-quality life apparently free from cancer, but the new year of 2006 had brought a devastating return of the disease. Rati passed away at the age of four years, just two months before Abby and Brenda visited Kenya.

It was for those two—her father and Rati—that Abby was here now. Neither of them could know what they had started, but Abby felt sure both would be proud, pleased with what she and her companions were doing and as delighted at the broad interest.

Brenda had been more than shocked; she had been amazed at the crowd of people who turned out to hear her speak. Even more memorable was the reaction of the cashier at the Nakumatt grocery store, which will stay with Brenda forever. On their second day in Kisumu, the woman caught sight of the T-shirts that Brenda, Abby, and Brian wore. She paused in mid-swipe, a carton of milk poised above the scanner while she read the caption (in Swahili) accompanying the unusual image of the afflicted child:

A white glow in a child's eye could be a sign of cancer.
If your child's eye looks like the photograph,
make sure a medical doctor checks both eyes urgently.
Untreated, children's eye cancer is fatal,
but when diagnosed early it is very curable.
Don't be slow. Help your child to be a survivor!

She read it once, twice, and then a third time before lifting her eyes from the message and asking the first of what was to be a barrage of questions. All around them, traffic in the grocery store stopped as people turned to listen. Mothers holding the hands of small children listened intently, seeking answers to questions of their own. The fire of awareness was set, interest kindling in the eyes of Kenyan parents.

"You know," Abby said as they left Nakumatt some time later with their purchases, "it might be worth seeing if we can persuade Nakumatt to put up posters in their stores, with the same message as the T-shirts. People are so interested . . ."

Brenda nodded, "Why not?"

Several weeks later, Brian, wearing a plain red shirt, and Abby, wearing a light jacket to cover her T-shirt, met with the operations manager of Nakumatt at their Nairobi headquarters. They were ushered into the manager's office, and smiling with polite disinterest, the man offered them a seat at his wide imposing desk.

When the pleasantries had passed, Abby drew out a laminated photo of the same image that graced the front of her concealed T-shirt. She slid it across the desk, asking, "What do you think is wrong with this child's eye?" The manager glanced at the picture, shrugged, and pushed it back.

"The child has eye cancer," Abby exclaimed simply as she removed her jacket, to reveal her T-shirt. The manager swept up the laminated photo and studied it hard, incredulous at the totally unexpected answer. The pair of visitors held his full attention for the next forty-five minutes, and when they finally left, it was with the promise that posters would be put up in every Nakumatt store across Kenya for a period of six months.

With help from Rati's father and others, the message was translated into many languages. Multiple translations of the poster and T-shirt could be used around the world to spread the word about curable childhood cancer!

The T-shirts were a success; posters were in production. There were no words to describe how well the campaign was going. The team was overjoyed by their success.

As Brenda's stay in Kenya drew close to an end, she and Abby took time to visit a young girl whose tumour had claimed her right eye. Her name was Lindah and, unlike Abby, her socket had not been filled by a prosthetic eye.

Lindah sat quietly on Brenda's lap with her family and friends in the living room of their tiny mud-walled home, three hours' drive from Kisumu. She spoke no English but understood that the visitors were here somehow because of her.

Abby naturally gravitated towards Lindah. She wanted to connect with the little girl, to share something important with her as another survivor. Without fuss or ceremony, Abby slipped her prosthetic eye out. She was aware of the silence—an audible reaction to this sudden revelation that she too had a "special eye." She and Lindah sat across from one another and she could almost feel the little girl's grin spreading. At last, she wasn't the only one missing an eye. Until then, Lindah had felt that other children and their parents treated her differently, fearing or just not understanding the empty eye socket and drooping lid. Those children now stood at the doorway to the house, peering in for a sight of the foreign visitors, and to hear what they had to say.

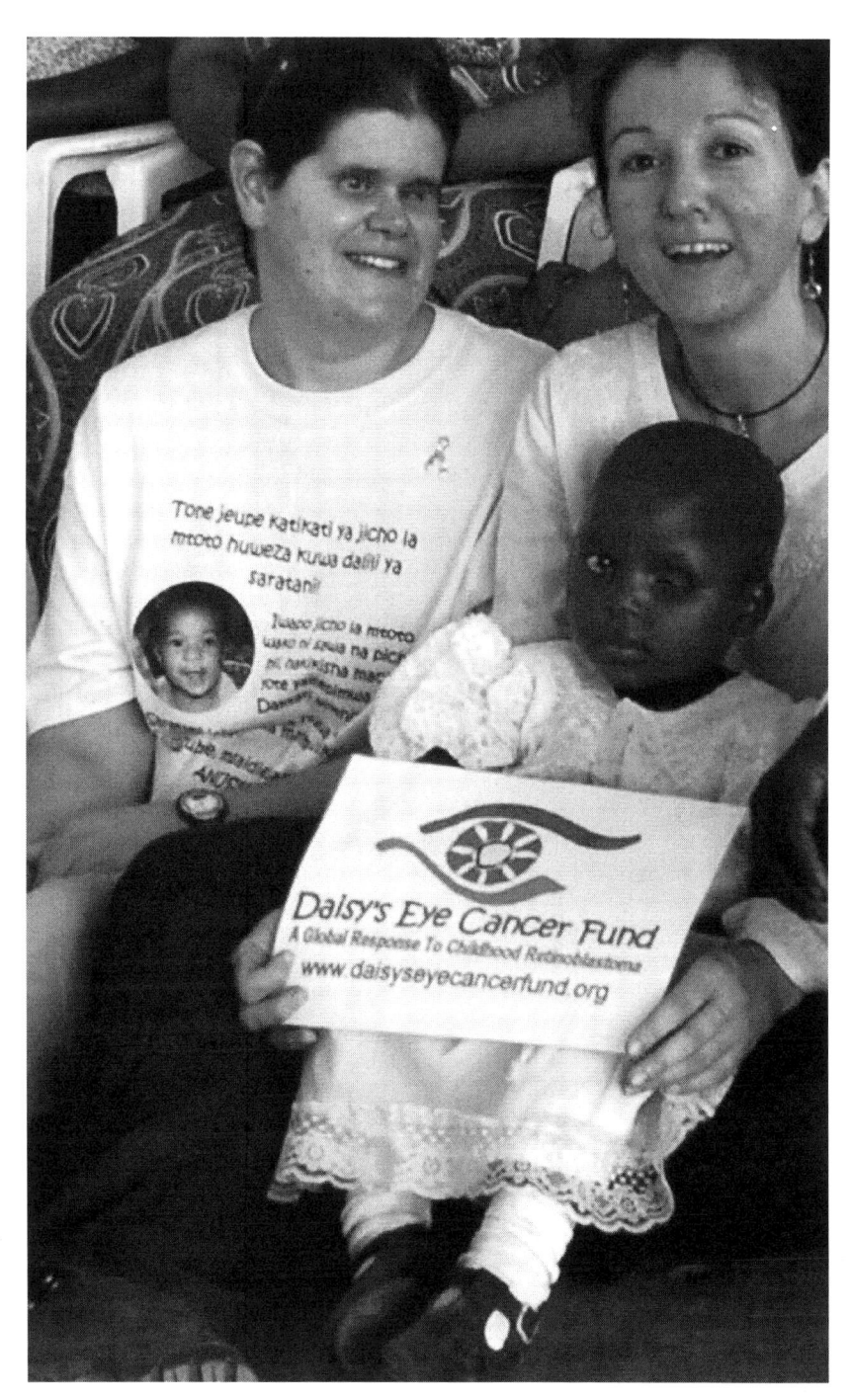

Abby, Lindah, and friend

The little living room was filled with murmurs, of shock, surprise, amazement, and relief. Abby smiled and reached across the table to take Lindah's hand. It was small and cool and it squeezed hers in gratitude. Maybe, just maybe, the people who had seen Abby remove her eye would understand a little and accept a lot more. She kept company with the child for the rest of the afternoon as the entire village gathered to learn about and understand Lindah's cancer.

The first phase of the pilot project was complete after one eventful week of unbelievable progress in Kisumu. Brian, Brenda, and Abby had much to discuss as they drove to Nairobi at the end of Brenda's first visit to Kenya.

Brenda gazed out of the window as her plane rolled down the runway. It seemed too big and too slow to lift off from the ground, to make it into the air, but the nose angled up, the wheels lifted off the tarmac and tucked up into the belly of the plane. As the vast expanse of Africa opened up below, Brenda marvelled at how the seemingly impossible can quickly take flight and reach new horizons.

Far below, Brian and Abby turned away from Jomo Kenyatta International Airport towards more meetings and steady progress. As he wove a path through the heavy noonday traffic, a tune came to Brian's lips. "I'm leaving on a jet plane. Don't know when I'll be back again . . ." Though the time and the place were uncertain, he was certain of one thing: The two remarkable women with whom he had shared this momentous week would return time and again to Kenya, and their campaign would take off as easily as the plane just departed.

Since that short visit three years ago, Brenda and Abby have returned to Kenya three times, and the NGO "Daisy's Eye Cancer Fund—Kenya" has been established with the mission of securing optimal care for all children and families affected by retinoblastoma in Kenya. The Kenyan National Retinoblastoma Strategy was launched in September 2008 to work towards this goal. Involving seventy medical professionals and patients from across Kenya, the strategy has introduced national awareness campaigns to help achieve early diagnosis, and created family support initiatives to assist families after diagnosis. Evidence-based protocols and guidelines for retinoblastoma are being developed for Kenya's resource-limited setting, and a national pathology service has been launched to enable appropriate post-operative care.

The campaign that began with a T-shirt in 2006 has truly taken flight.

Susan Croft is a student of English and history at Queen's University in Kingston, where she is an active member of the rock-climbing club and the Kingston Writers' Circle.

The Texture of a Word

Ian G. Dorward

I'm surprised to see him wearing street clothes, sitting on the side of the bed. After rounding on him each morning for three days, the surreal 5:00 a.m. haze pouring through the window, my conception of this man has become inextricably tied to disposable nylon pants and a bare chest traversed by IV tubing. Seeing him now sitting upright, wearing a beige striped shirt and khaki slacks, I find myself disoriented. Quickly I check my patient list to ensure that I'm in the right room: 13456, Bed A, Mr. Powell. Yep. Right patient, right room. I say hello.

He greets me with the same cheery grin his face has borne the past several mornings—only this time he doesn't have to struggle through drowsiness to force it out. The smile comes from a warm place, and I want to sit beside him on the bed. Maybe put my arm around his shoulders. Mostly I just think I should touch him—a hand on his elbow, or even gloved fingers on the question-mark-shaped incision arching across his shaved scalp. Instead I fidget, totter on my feet, pat the pockets of my white coat, cross my arms. I try to smile, but not too much.

He knows why I'm here. He knows that it's not to say hello or to perform a routine neurologic exam in the middle of the afternoon. I think for a moment about launching into my exam anyhow, asking him his name and the date, checking to see if he can name a few items in my pockets and repeat back to me, "No ifs, ands, or buts." But why? He's a retired college physics professor, and probably still smarter than me, even after having a four-centimetre tumour cut from his left frontal lobe. His mental status is no more in question than mine; at least he's slept more than four hours each of the past five nights. Why bother? The subterfuge would cheat us both.

So I begin.

I couch my words in preface, gauging the appropriate degree of medical jargon to employ. I think to myself, Would he want it straight out? Or is he the type of man who wants this news swaddled in hope, cradled gently in reassurance? I see a frown on his face as I get tangled in my words, tripping where I had wanted to tiptoe. "Just tell me," he says, clutching his pants above his knees, crinkling the fabric into bunches in his palms. "You've been great, you know, explaining to me diseases and treatments in terms a layperson can understand. Not to mention cutting the damn thing out. I've appreciated everything you've done for me—I can't thank you enough. Don't spoil it by pussyfooting around. Tell me. Is it a glioblastoma?"

He looks at me frankly, his eyes unblinking, his expression washed of content. It's just a face, on just a man. And he wants just the truth.

"Yes, it is," I say. "The pathologists have finished their report, and they say that it's a glioblastoma." My voice trails off with the last word, so much that I wonder if it was audible. Reflexively I say it again, "Glioblastoma."

Inadvertently I had framed the word. Bracketed, standing alone, it faces him in bold strokes and stark contrasts. He stares at it, hanging on the wall somewhere beyond my left shoulder; there, in its sharp lines and dark hues, he sees his sixty-five preceding years in dull relief, trailing off in the distance like a shadow at dusk. Standing in the foreground are twelve more months—fifteen at best—punctuated by chemotherapy and radiation and lost hair and cognitive difficulties and intractable nausea and expressive aphasia and steroid psychosis and a re-operation and implanted chemotherapy wafers and an infected wound and another operation and a cerebral abscess and IV antibiotics and deep venous thrombosis and an inferior vena cava filter and swallowing dysfunction and a G-tube and hospice. And a race between pain and narcotics, the former the certain victor.

His right hand slowly moves from his pants leg to his pocket and produces a white handkerchief. He carefully unfolds it. It is old, washed many times, and frayed slightly at the edges. A part of me wishes I knew what it felt like, what sensation the well-laundered cotton weave would leave on the fingertips. He drapes it over his hand and uses it to dab at his forehead. Afterwards he drops his hand to his lap, and the handkerchief lies in soft rumples. It looks strangely elegant, splayed out over his fingers like some liturgical shroud.

He looks up at me once, briefly. "Thank you, doctor," he says, "for everything."

Then the handkerchief is crumpled in his fist. As I walk out of the room I glance once more over my shoulder; I see the handkerchief cast upon the floor. Above it his feet swing up onto the end of the bed and one crosses over the other, his soles facing towards the wall. He stays that way for several hours, and I continue my day.

Ian Dorward is a neurosurgery resident. He likes to spend his rare out-of-hospital moments writing. This happens to be his first publication.

Table of Unidentified Contents
A Portfolio of Intaglio Prints

Doug Guildford

I have been living in downtown Toronto for the past twenty-five years. Toronto is my social and cultural base. The diversity, here, feeds, supports, and reassures me.

Concurrently, however, I have returned each year to my place of origin, the Atlantic coast of Nova Scotia, where I inhabit the amphibious zone between the tides; a quasi-land of shapeshifting, addition, subtraction, and flux.

This is my wilderness area. It is my reference point with the natural world and my creative source.

My art practice is firmly rooted in drawing. Drawing works for me, both as a language for problem solving and as a tool for self-reflection.

I see the drawings and the prints as notations or lab notes, a compulsive kind of journal entry, and, perhaps, a distillation of accumulated knowledge.

I am continuing to develop an ongoing and extensive body of drawing and print-work based on my evolving "glossary" of graphic terms (an automatic shorthand for my take on the universe). This language is based upon my experience and observation of life forms at the edge of my native shore. It is a calligraphy that wanders suggestively between male and female and lays claim to the ambiguous terrain of the intertidal zone.

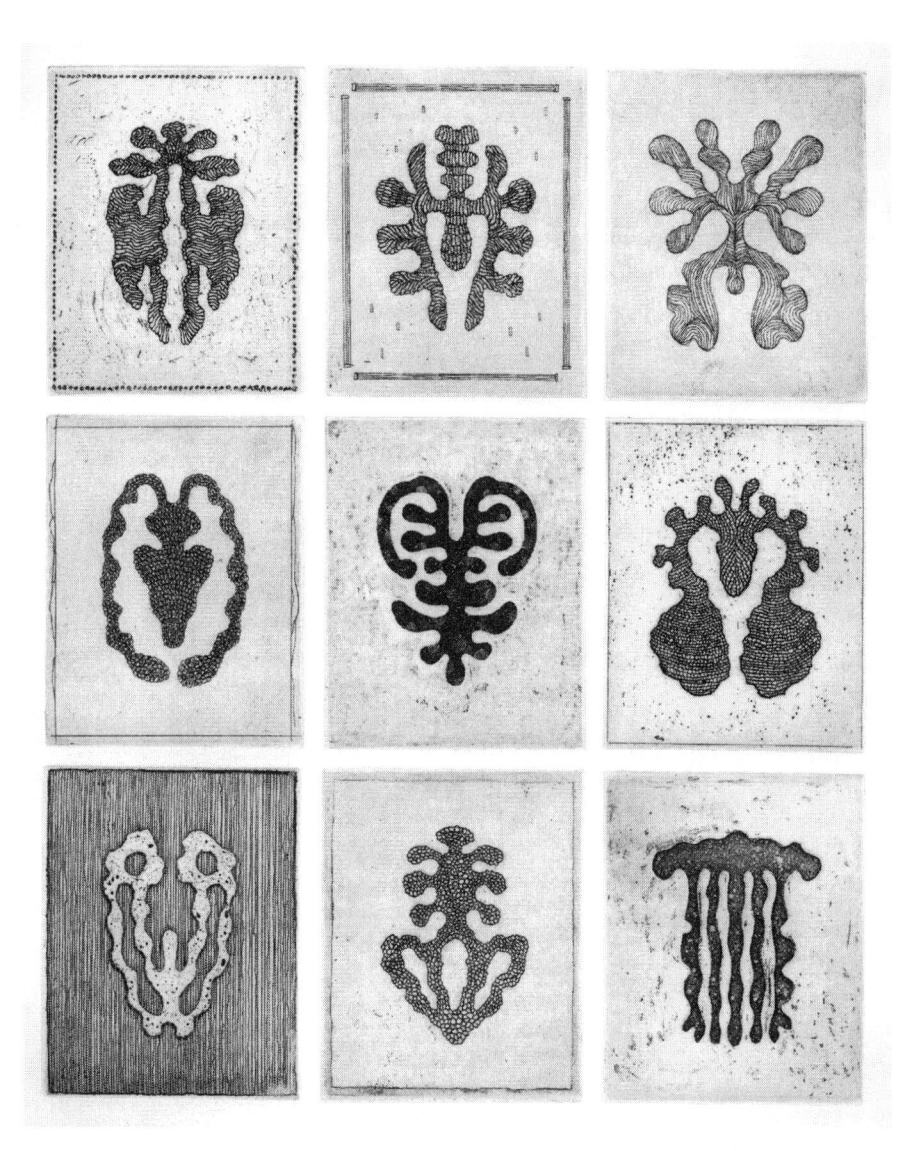

Spring Thaw (2004). Etching, 32 x 26 cm

Doug Guildford prints at Open Studio, teaches sessionally, and is represented in Toronto by Edward Day Gallery. His work is showcased globally over the Internet by the Centre for Contemporary Canadian Art (www.ccca.ca).

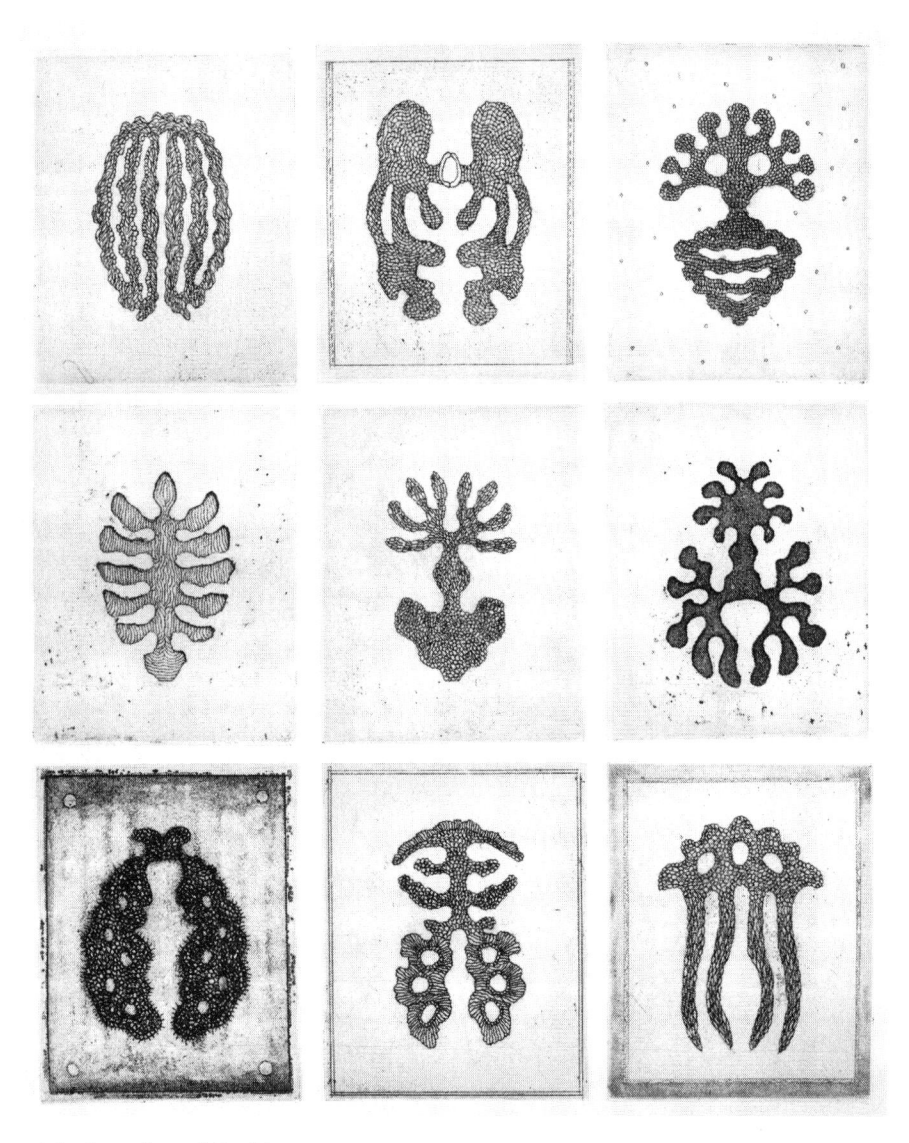

Mid Winter (2004). Etching, 32 x 26 cm

Figuring the Ground

Pam Hall

Pam Hall spent two years as the first artist-in-residence in the Faculty of Medicine at Memorial University, St. John's. Her work there in a variety of media can be viewed as attentive research into how doctors "learn the body"—see it, touch it, to feel it, and know it.

Designed to create and sustain dialogue and conversation with both the learning and clinical community within the school and Health Sciences Center, her work consistently invited response and interaction. Figuring the Ground is a series of drawings of the hands of some of Hall's student collaborators. It is populated with echoes of their voices as they spoke about their aspirations as physicians. It is on loan and display at the medical school. A detailed report on the medical school residency can be found at http://www.med.mun.ca/artistinresidence/.

Pam Hall's most recent major exhibition was New Readings in Female Anatomy, at venues across Canada. The catalogue for that installation will be published by Carleton University Art Gallery, Ottawa, and The Rooms, St. John's.

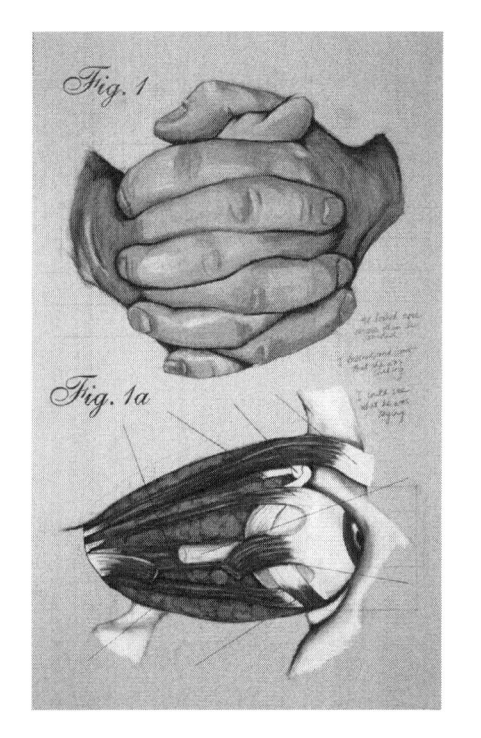

Fig. 1

Fig. 1a

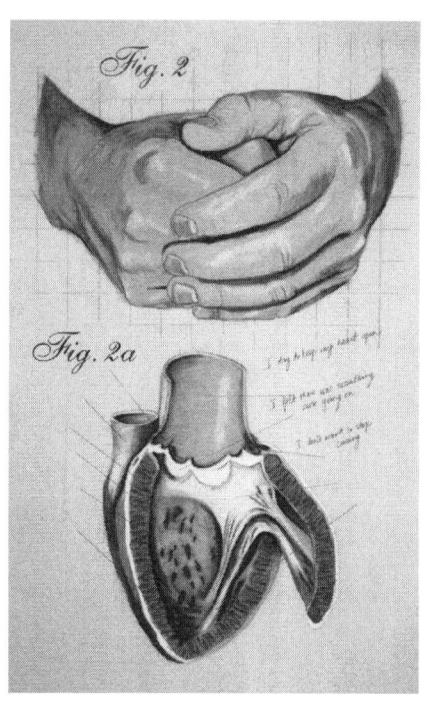

Fig. 2

Fig. 2a

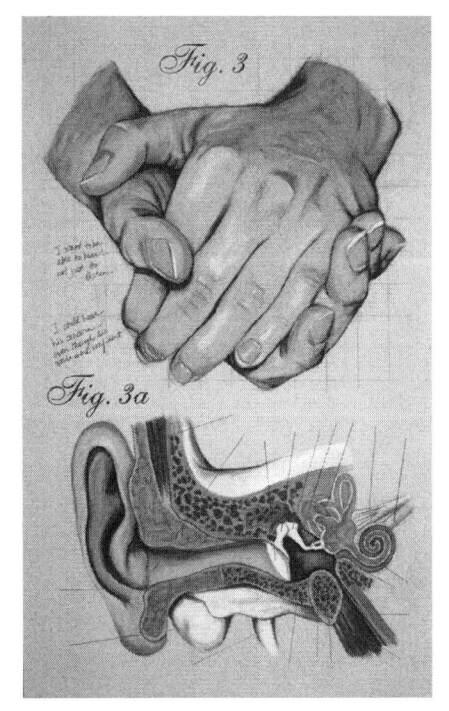

Fig. 3

Fig. 3a

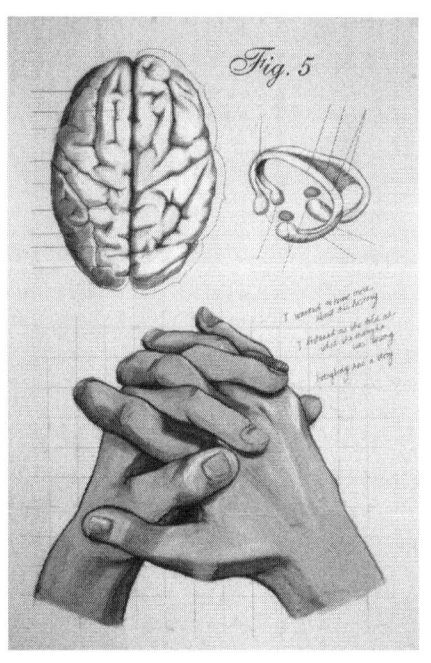

Fig. 5

258

Refugees in Southeast Asia[1]

J. David Holbrook

At sunrise a week later, having revamped the apartment and registered the children at school, Lauretta waved as I left the apartment for Kalang, the port for Kuala Lumpur. It was hard to leave so soon after Lauretta and the children had arrived, but travelling was a crucial part of the job.

I was the only passenger in a Malaysian police launch, on my way to international waters, the sun hot on my back even at this early hour. A burly Malay policeman stepped back from the front of the launch and shoved a red arm band in my face.

"Put this on! Wear it at all times! This is your pass. We will be in a security zone." As a diplomat, I was being offered no favours.

The launch blasted off from the jetty, the wake flooding the numerous dugouts and their occupants, fishing in the shallows of the Kalang harbour.

I watched as the Malay fishermen struggled to right their boats and bail them out with their rusty tin cans. There were no angry gestures. Flocks of screeching seagulls circled and zoomed in on fish the locals couldn't retrieve. Navigating the colossal container ships, we finally came into the Straits of Malacca, leaving behind the stench of rotting fish and garbage.

The salt sea smell in the straits was a relief but the noticeable swell was not. The rising sun on the waves at the front of the launch painted

---

1. Chapter 2 of *A Diplomatic Doctor*, published by iUniverse, 2005

the water with green and gold highlights as we cut through it. Anchored in the distance was a rusted, sickly looking freighter: my destination.

The *Hai Hong* ("Sea Breeze" in Chinese) was a floating piece of scrap, which had secretly left Singapore and anchored in the estuary of the Saigon River near the town of Vung Tau, south of Saigon, in October 1978. There, it took a load of 2,510 desperate people willing to pay US$3200 or sixteen pieces of gold to leave Vietnam. Children were supposedly half-price.

The cost was worth it to many in South Vietnam's middle classes. They were facing re-education camps and hard labour, separation from their families, and, at worst, long prison terms for supporting the losing side during the war. The final blow was that these families were then obliged to move out of Saigon to "new economic zones"—a euphemism for a plot of jungle where new communities were to be established. They comprised the part of Vietnamese society that could not and would not support a unified Vietnam under a "socialist" regime governing from Hanoi in the north—the traditional rival of Saigon in the south. There were no longer positions for teachers, doctors, or lawyers in Saigon, which were now all taken by northern newcomers.

The syndicate responsible for the *Hai Hong* was made up of Vietnamese officials, Singaporean promoters, and the Hong Kong owners of the salvaged freighter. They made a profit of four to five million dollars on this voyage alone. Trafficking in human lives had become an easy way to make money, if you didn't give a damn about what happened to them.

As the *Hai Hong* left Vietnam and moved into the South China Sea, neighbouring countries were alerted to its presence. All had refugee camps overflowing from earlier arrivals. A year earlier another supposedly scrapped freighter, the *Southern Cross*, had floated into Indonesian waters and dumped 1,200 refugees for the government of Indonesia to house. The *Hai Hong* was going to be forbidden to land anywhere in Southeast Asia. After weeks of drifting back and forth at sea, refused entry over and over again and battered by a typhoon, the diesel engines failed, leaving the 1,600 ton freighter drifting off the Malaysian coast.

The United Nations High Commission for Refugees appealed to Canada, and others, to share the responsibility for the *Hai Hong*'s cargo as a humanitarian gesture. When finally an agreement was reached to launch a relief mission, Malaysia would still not allow the *Hai Hong* to enter its waters. The processing had to be done at sea. As part of that team I was responsible for the health of the refugees bound for Canada.

As the launch approached, I could see the rusted orange hull looming over me. A squiggly white strip painted without care, white paint dripping into the rusty black, stretched from bow to stern, with the new name *Hai Hong* printed on both sides of the bow, in white. Streams of dirty bilge water poured out of holes in the hull and splashed into the sea beside me. Was this from the engine room? Was this the toilets draining? Toilets? There probably weren't any. Three decks teemed with bodies pushing against the rail—men, women, and children of all ages, shouting and waving banners:

"FEED US!"

"TAKE US TO YOUR COUNTRY!"

"WE WANT TO GO TO AMERICA!"

"NO FOOD! NO WATER!"

I felt sick with horror and disgust at what was happening in front of my eyes. Could these people have expected this when they paid their money? Would they still think it worthwhile? The sight of this mass of desperate humanity shouting and screaming was overwhelming.

The police launch was now circling the Malaysian Navy frigate already at the scene. It kept the *Hai Hong* from going anywhere. The launch finally came alongside and I was waved to the front to transfer to the larger Navy vessel. Five Canadian immigration officers stationed in Malaysia were already on board.

"Welcome aboard, David. We sure need a doctor," quipped a smiling Dick Williams.

I tried to stand still on the deck of the frigate to get my balance back. Over the side of the *Hai Hong* dangled a rotten wooden ladder with rungs missing, pieces of frayed rope filling the gaps.

"OK Holbrook, you're the doctor, you go first."

The ladder thudded back and forth against the hull. It stretched from just below the first deck railing to three feet above my head. By standing on the steel railings of the frigate, I could just reach the first rung, with a boost from my compatriots. I didn't have much choice and so rather than think about it, I grabbed the end of the ladder. Careful not to fall through the holes where rungs once were, I hauled myself up the side to the first deck. I was met by a cheering mob of people who grabbed my arms and pulled me over the rusty uneven railing onto the deck.

The stench of sweat, stale urine, and feces was nauseating. I was now jammed into the mass of people, moving as one, as the ship swayed. I was tugged away from the rail by an unseen arm and found myself closer to the centre of the deck. There was a noticeable listing, sending pots and various containers sliding past me. I watched a giant tub of thick brown slop slip by without tipping.

I suddenly realized that there were jagged holes in the deck above, allowing excrement and garbage to drop from deck to deck. No wonder the spot I was trying to stand on was so slimy. I pushed through the crowd to the port side, thinking there might be more air there.

Four people were laid out on the deck with filthy sheets over them. There was no movement and only the tops of their heads were visible. I asked the nearest person, motioning at the four bodies, "Are they sick?"

"Oh yes, sir!" said a woman, hauling me by the elbow to their side. She gingerly pulled back each sheet. Was the odour the sweet smell of rotting flesh, or the filthy sheets? I crouched beside the first of the four.

Under the sheet was a teenager with third-degree burns, grey patches roughly six inches wide on her shoulders and chest, oozing and peeling around the edges. The sheet—her only covering from the waist up—stuck to the wounds as I tried to peel it off to expose the entire burn. She wouldn't look at me, or at the burn.

I didn't have any instruments to remove the dead skin or any dressings to cover it properly.

"Is there anyone here who speaks English?" I said.

The woman beside me nodded.

"Please tell this girl that we are going to get bandages for her burns and clean sheets."

"Can I still go to Canada?" moaned the teenager.

I smiled, looking back, surprised to hear her talking. "Yes, I'm sure we'll find a way."

Next was an elderly man with a crinkly face, papery skin, and a toothless grin . . . or was it a grimace? What looked like a jagged puncture wound was surrounded by grey, burned, dead skin in the centre of his abdomen. Surprisingly, there seemed to be little blood loss around the wound. I held his arm and took a closer look. It was hard to tell if it was only superficial, but surely he would be dead if his bowel had been punctured. He tried to lift his head to see what I was looking at. I didn't want to touch the wound as my hands were filthy, although I don't suppose I would have introduced any bacteria he didn't already have.

"Boiler blew, Doctor."

I held his arm as I explained to the woman beside him how to clean the wounds.

The middle-aged woman lying next to him had red blotchy burns on her neck. She could not move her head without grimacing. There wasn't the dead, greyish hue of third-degree burns, but instead weepy, red patches. It would be a nasty scar, but she would heal better than the other two.

Finally, the teenager next to her had red-streaked burns across the tops of both feet that stretched up his legs. He seemed quite blasé about it all, but obviously could not stand up or move his feet. An antibiotic ointment was needed.

Propped up nearby was a young woman with her right ankle protruding at an odd angle.

"Not much doubt about that fracture," I said to myself, thinking finally I had something relatively simple to deal with. All that could be done was to find a piece of wood for a splint until we could get it X-rayed and set properly.

"Is there a nurse in this group?" I asked the woman helping with the sheets.

"I'm a nurse, Doctor," she replied.

There was a provision for taking a small number of ill and injured refugees off the ship. These four would qualify.

"I am going to send you bandages and a splint. Please do the best that you can to dress the wounds and we will try to move these people to shore soon."

The old man tried again to raise his head and held his arm up to shake my hand.

I was swarmed by people on all sides trying to grab me to get assurances that they could get off this floating hell-hole and go to Canada. Neatly printed, pleading letters in Vietnamese, French, and English were stuffed into all of my pockets. I smiled without agreeing to do anything and made my way back to the ladder.

Going back down the side was worse than going up. The ladder slammed back and forth with the swell, out then in, crunching against the side of the freighter. I didn't want to get my hand caught between the side of the ladder and the hull, so I moved down slowly, trying to time each step with the motion of the ship. I breathed a sigh of relief as I jumped from the last step onto the deck of the frigate.

I jotted down a list of necessities for the nurse on board. I wondered where I'd collect it all. The captain of the frigate joined us as we set up a table for the interviews on the deck under the canopy shielding the Bofors anti-aircraft gun.

"Captain, would it be possible to have some sheets and burn dressings for four patients on the freighter?" I asked, looking him in the eye. I bit my lip, hoping for a positive reply.

"Yes, we can help with that," said the captain, solving the problem easily.

"We'll interview refugees claiming to have relatives in Canada first," announced Dick Williams, the leader of the immigration officers. "David, you'll have to do your medical examination on the other side of the gun, then send them on to Bill, who will try to do a police report. Sorry Bill, you're going to be in the sun."

I smiled to myself, wondering what good a "police report" was going to be. Would anybody with a police record be honest under these circumstances?

"How on earth are we going to get them off the *Hai Hong* and then back on again after the interview?" I asked.

"We interviewed a spokesperson for the refugees while you were on board and he has chosen an individual on each of the three decks who can speak English. That person will get two people from each deck at the top and bottom of the ladder to help move the people on and off the ship. The spokesman will be the overall organizer of the procedure," explained Dick. "It's his task to coordinate the interview process, deciding who is to be interviewed on the frigate."

"We're going to have to stop if the sea gets any rougher. We can't afford any catastrophes."

Dick continued, "Lists are being prepared and submitted to the captain, who in turn will tell us how many he will allow on the deck of the frigate each hour, from dawn to dusk."

Tall and gaunt, the *Hai Hong*-appointed leader was the first person down the ladder with the initial list of interviewees in his hand.

"I am Dat Luu Phuoc." He put out his hand and smiled. I watched in amazement as he navigated the ladder with ease. He spoke fluent English and agreed to translate for us on the Navy vessel. We went over the procedures with him.

Phuoc's wife and five daughters had disappeared at sea or were in another refugee camp. The details were neatly written on a folded piece of paper and stuffed in my pocket. He wanted me to look in the camps for them.

Day one was over at sunset. We fell exhausted into the launch for the trip back to Port Kalang before total darkness. Looking back at the *Hai Hong*, I could only see the vague outline of the black hulk in the water with a few candles flickering on each deck.

Dawn to dusk. Dawn to dusk. For a week it was the same seafood dinner, the same grimy roach-infested room in the Port View Hotel with the flashing red neon sign outside my window that made it seem even hotter. In my narrow bed I twisted around, flipped my pillow, and kicked off the sheet. I was unable to put the thoughts of the previous day out of my mind.

The interviews were makeshift at best. Applicants ranged in age from two weeks old—born during the voyage—to eighty-two years. To get so many down the deepest ladder and back up was a major logistical feat. I examined each person with my hands and a stethoscope, attempting to rule out tuberculous lungs. The refugees should have received extra health credits for having the agility to manage the ladder as it swayed precariously back and forth against the hull.

The youngest of the refugees was virtually a newborn.

"When was the baby born? Is he your first child?" I asked his mother.

"Yes, he was born twenty days ago," she replied, though I could barely hear her over the screaming of the thin but clear-eyed infant. The baby didn't look sick. The umbilical cord, however, was a soggy mess, still attached with no sign of drying up. I couldn't pull it for fear of making it worse.

Tetanus? There didn't seem to be any muscle tightness other than that caused by the yelling. There was no question that he was able to open his mouth and swing his arms around. The only case of tetanus I had ever seen was two weeks ago in one of the camps—a baby with an infected umbilical cord. Could this be another case of the same thing? I dressed it as well as I could, cleaning away as much of the grunge around the cord as possible, and used the antibiotic ointment the captain had given me.

I made a mental note to get some anti-tetanus toxin from the US Embassy doctors, who were always lifesavers when all else failed.

Being the only one with a camera and extra film, I took the seventy passport pictures. It was soon working like clockwork.

"Please come here and lie on the couch while I examine you and go there and smile because I'm going to take your picture. No arguments allowed."

There were none. There was, however, much apprehension.

I doubted that any of the oldsters had ever had their photograph taken. In Asia, it was thought that a photo could take away part of your soul that could never be retrieved. In this case, was it a fair price to pay for freedom and a new life? The backdrop for these mug shots—an anti-aircraft turret and flapping khaki canvas—no doubt added a nice touch to the travel permits.

The transfer to the airport in Kuala Lumpur from the *Hai Hong* began with the burns victims. They were lowered over the side on borrowed stretchers, each of us manning a rope and praying that the rusted railing would not give way.

As the sun set on the final day of the *Hai Hong* for me, I looked at all those still waiting, standing by the rail at the top of the flimsy ladder, softly weeping, wringing their hands and waiting and waiting as the launch sped away.

Having graduated from UofT, David Holbrook practised family medicine prior to joining the Canadian government as a foreign service officer, with postings in Trinidad, Singapore, the United Kingdom, Mexico, and India. He died shortly after publication of this piece in Ars Medica's Fifth Anniversary Edition.

Mid-winter Night

Jill Leahman

I've invited the cadaver over, asked him
to tuck entrails back into the cavity
because the puppy likes to grab things
and run with them. This would be
a problem, I explain. I tell him
I need a muse and you are as close
as I've come, though by no means
are you traditional. I thought we might
have a glass of wine, listen to Norah Jones,
talk about the state of the garden.
I tell him about my dissertation, how
the due day looms. He just shakes his head,
hollowed cheeks catching the light.

His face dips in and out of shadow.
I tell him about catalogues, pop-up ads, commercials
all hawking an easier, more beautiful life.
He just listens, not saying much. His life is
unremarkable these days. Students work on him,
lifting away layers to study the inner workings
of a body hard-used. He has time to listen.
Outside the front door rhododendron leaves
curl into themselves as if they were trying to find
some warmth on a February night. I take his hand
hardened with chemicals and holding nothing,
thank him for his visit and send him back. He says
the cold is comforting, says he doesn't remember
how a warm body feels anymore.

Summer Party

In the yard people gather in twos and threes,
heads bent, leaning into one another.
Here the scent of rosemary
lingers in the air, released by the weight of feet,
people dancing, arms over heads,
dipping in time, or not in time, to the music.

This is what I miss most, says the cadaver,
the possibility of love. A man and woman sit on the step,
talking, their thighs barely touching. She leans
against his shoulder, laughing and teasing.
The cadaver says the smells will stay with them,
filling a place in memory, so that each time a part of her will remember
these laughing moments. What will remind you of me, he asks.

I have no answer ready. I look up at the sky, clouds
like ghosts. The smell of smoke, pale glow of mushrooms
in the wood, amber of scotch, a cool hand,
closed eyes. I ask if he is leaving and if so when.
He says, the moon has risen full, tells me to watch
for the owl at night. It will guide you
back. Still the dancers dance, swaying in the dark.
all of it too much, the scents of this world, the laughter,
the thighs brushing against each other in the dark.

I finally have his answer.
The moonlight, I tell him. See here, it dances over my arm
and there you are running in my veins.

Jill Karle Leahman lives, teaches writing, and writes in Charlottesville, VA, at the base of the Blue Ridge. Recent publications include Tough Times, Eclipse, Blueline. *Work is forthcoming in* Poetry Motel, Comstock Review, *and* PMS.

On Pathography

Robert Maunder

Thirty years ago, when I subscribed to MAD magazine, there was a recurring section that featured Very Thin Books, such as *On Morality* by Richard M. Nixon. A few years later, in university, while navigating the undergraduate course that marked the shortest distance between high school and an MD, and therefore led more sensible students to divide all bits of learning into categories of "might be on the exam" and "superfluous," I felt the distracting pull to obtain a liberal education. I didn't. However, I did appreciate finding Kenneth Rexroth's *Classics Revisited*, which offered a taste of what I had missed and introduced me to both the *Epic of Gilgamesh* and the idea of a short bookshelf. Although I was grateful, even then I could tell that the short bookshelf, like the parlour game Desert Island Collection of Books or Records, is impossible to get just right, and is the easy victim of snobbery and concessions to accepted taste. Still, all these years later I still enjoy desert island collections and 100-best lists. A short bookshelf may be shallow, or may be merely introductory, but, if compiled in good faith, it is a personal statement, a Rorschach of taste, experience, and idiosyncrasy.

This essay could be a Very Thin Book. I have never been seriously ill, which may disqualify me for my task. But my intention is not a Thin Book but a short bookshelf of pathography. The word refers to illness narratives, the genre of literature composed of stories of being sick. I had never heard of pathography, until I started (post-MAD, post-Rexroth, post-MD) to collect first-hand accounts of being sick as a teaching aid. I teach psychiatric residents to care for the medically ill. Descriptions of being sick, although not on the exam, seemed a very useful way for young doctors to learn what the person who they are trying to care for is going through. The best teaching aid would be to make the doctors sick, at least for a while. But making all your students sick virtually rules out the possibility of teaching awards and promotion. Second-best is to listen carefully to the stories of a thousand or so people whose lives have been changed by illness. For the sake of efficiency we move to Plan C—to read well-written accounts of what it is like to be sick, to suffer, and to face death. Along the way I learned that these stories form a genre and that it has a name.

At the start, I imagined that literary accounts of being sick would be hard to find. The whole set might fit on a short bookshelf. In fact, there are thousands of them. The themes that emerge from these stories, however, are relatively few. This is my list: death and dying, dealing with doctors, sex and matters of the flesh, loss, monotony and fatigue, pain, aloneness, uncertainty, meaning, and self-pity. It would be sensible to add triumph to the list, although I tend to avoid triumphant stories of illness, which often seem too stretched across the imperative of victory to resonate as an actual experience of a complex trouble. The best pathographies, like the best novels and poems, I suppose, describe life with subtlety, contradiction, emotion, depth, beauty, and banality. But it helps to read the best.

What about the worst? I have my prejudices. Susan Sontag has alerted us to the pernicious effects of the metaphors that describe illness. Of course, metaphor cannot be avoided—it would be awful to try—but certain metaphors of illness come very easily and yield little in return: illness is a battle, for example. The battle metaphor is often telegraphed by the book's subtitle, a phrase that includes the words *survivor, beat, inspiring, triumph, uplifting,* or *battle*. Triumphant battles, however much they actually do convey an important part of the experience of being sick for many people, seem to me to be the expectation of the well, more likely to be received and lived up to (or not) by someone who is ill, than the authentic experience that emerges from living with disease. I am more convinced by Brant Frayne, who had a stroke and an aneurysm in his forties and wrote,

> I know that articles like this one, stories of people "cut down in their prime" are supposed to have happy endings, or at least a sense of promise. I'm sorry I can't end with a hallelujah moment, with a tri-

umph or even with catharsis. There is no possibility of victory, no pass or fail, no reason to think better times lie ahead. The test never ends. Ten years after the stroke, I wonder why I didn't die that day while on the table, and still often wish that I had. Even in my subconscious, I'm crippled; I've never had a dream in which I was whole again.[1]

My list of common themes suggests that existential truth is a more common nidus of reflection for the seriously ill writer than personal triumph. Illness is not different from life, in that sense, except that it rubs your face in it. Illness is the great destroyer of denial.

I'll take that back. The battle metaphor of destruction is not appropriate in this instance either. What serious illness does to denial is make it obvious. Young and healthy people are entitled to think that their lives matter, that they are not alone (except in their solipsistic divinity), and that they will live forever. For the very young it is almost inevitable. Even older people, if they are sensibly optimistic, underestimate the proximity of death. I heard an expert in these things say that, statistically, the probability that an adult will die before the year is up is 1 in 200. How many healthy people wake up in the morning contemplating those odds? But to have a life-threatening disease, to be too tired to participate, to be close to death, is to be in a condition where it strains credulity to believe that life is not finite, limited, and lonely. And for many, the point of it all becomes a point of contention. In one of the great pathographies, the book of Job, the silly rationalizations of the well are cast aside by Job who suffers with painful boils from head to foot. It is *not* true that he is ill because he has sinned, or that God only punishes the evil. It is incredible to frame his ailment as a test of faith, because he passes the test so many times and yet is not rewarded with relief. His suffering is arbitrary and pointless. My patients, who suffer much more than I do, teach me about patience, fortitude, redemption, and faith. But more often they teach me not to strain so hard to find some redemptive thing in a state of affairs that may in truth be of no good to anybody.

I have read that pain cannot be described, but I have also read Robert Mason Lee's description of the pain of Crohn's disease, and many people with this chronic intestinal condition have told me that he is exactly right:

What does Crohn's disease feel like? It feels like three processes at once. First, a mule is kicking you in the stomach. Second, some maniac is inflating your abdomen with a bicycle pump. Third, you are being impaled up the ass with a pointy stick. I suppose the sensation must compare with labour, as the pain comes in waves triggered by abdominal contractions. A better comparison would be an ectopic pregnancy, since the pain is also overlaid with distress and panic and a sense of something having gone terribly wrong. Still, all comparisons are odious. What it feels like most of all is that you are suddenly, and without warning, very, very sick.[2]

Patients nod their heads when I read that passage to them as if finally someone has captured their experience. Students laugh at the profanity, but they also get it. It is a description that conveys the experience of that particular pain very well to someone who has never felt it. It isn't impossible, but it takes a good writer.

The best writers of pathography to my mind are the ones who are curious and unashamed enough to write about what illness has done to their minds and preferences and relationships and thoughts in a way that convinces me that they are also just discovering this strange situation for the first time, sometimes with amazement. There is Tom Andrews's startled realization—as he describes with tortured humour his exchange with a dim Emergency Department intern who is assessing him while the hemophiliac writer absorbs the excruciating pain of bleeding into a joint—that he is trying to make the young man fall in love with him so that he will give him morphine. Or Anatole Broyard's assessment of his urologist's pretentious vocabulary: "I can't die with this man. He wouldn't understand what I was saying. I'm going to say something brilliant when I die."[3]

Broyard deserves an essay all to himself. One imagines from reading his prose that he would like that. He wrote a pathography that should be on any short bookshelf of the genre, *Intoxicated by My Illness*, while dying of prostate cancer. Although the short book is littered with nuggets of insight, what lingers for me a few years after reading it is an afterimage of the personality of the man who wrote it. I have read few other essays where the author is so completely alive and present in the text, in all his narcissistic, gleeful, annoying, contemplative splendour.

Which brings me to another version of the hope for redemption through illness—the idea that one lives more fully when faced with the crisis of the finite. This may be the existential version of the same sentimental dead end that insists on triumph as an outcome of adversity, but I find it more compelling. In a sense this idea is just the result of the cosmic supply–demand curve: less life = higher value. Ivan Illych discovers how badly he has lived his life—"It was all not the right thing"—in a bolt of insight just two hours before he dies. But talking to just a few people with unreasonably short prospects is enough to make clear that living more fully is not a necessary outcome of serious illness. Bitterness, fear, loneliness, tedium, frustration, and indifference are just as common. In fact, several illness narratives emphasize that tedium is an under-appreciated but central part of being sick, as Plath and Andrews respectively demonstrate:

> They have propped my head between the pillow and the sheet-cuff
> Like an eye between two white lids that will not shut.
> Stupid pupil, it has to take everything in.
> The nurses pass and pass, they are no trouble,
> They pass the way gulls pass inland on white caps,
> Doing things with their hands, one just the same as another,
> So it is impossible to tell how many there are.[4]

> The narcosis of television. Watching TV for hours is like taking a great deal of codeine when you have no pain. The more you take it, the more you develop a need for it that can never be satisfied. Like pain, watching TV for hours has no content. Unlike pain, it kills time. Which, as Ezra Pound said, is fine if you like your time dead.[5]

Illness rubs your face in it. It rubs your face in the limits of life, in our reliance on one another, in astonishing personal strengths and appalling weakness, in the arbitrariness of events. Illness is a test of relationship, of values, and of faith—but as Job teaches us, it is a test that, once passed, continues nonetheless.

Susan Sontag, even while shucking off the metaphors of illness by cataloguing them, provides another metaphor of her own. Illness is a foreign land that most of us visit temporarily as tourists and then return home. It is another matter to make it your new home. What can those of us who have a passport but no intention of relocating do with our friends and family in the Land of Sick? Can we understand at all? Robert Lee Mason describes everyone's first inclination, to offer advice about things of which they have no understanding:

> I do my best to forgive these people their helpful instinct, because I understand the desire to heal as one of the primal social imperatives ... It's just that very few of us are good at healing, or tendering advice.
>
> What I have found, instead, is that just about everyone is good at offering comfort. I have had the hands of compassion laid upon me by doctors, nurses, ambulance attendants, the women in my life, friends, the wives of friends, complete strangers in bus terminals. When it comes to offering solace, people have a natural ability which transcends social place or relationships. We just give, naturally, of ourselves to those in need. One small consolation of having such a painful illness is the many opportunities it allows others to show kindness; the one great reassurance is how seldom I have been disappointed. And I have accepted compassion willingly in my life, knowing that I am a small, cracked vessel for others to pour in their love.[6]

And why do people write about being sick at all? In an age of singer-songwriters, celebrity tell-alls, dawn-to-dusk Oprah and Rosie and Jerry Springer, reality TV on every channel, and Internet diaries by the famous and the never-to-be famous, it may be a question that no longer needs to be asked. Maybe all just need to tell their story. But I think it is different to tell a story about being ill. It is more like being, maybe, a traveller returned from Sontag's foreign land (or sending a dispatch from deep within its borders), who needs to communicate an extraordinary, almost incomprehensible experience to listeners, who need just as badly to understand it. I think Broyard gets it right.

> What a critically ill person needs above all is to be understood. Dying is a misunderstanding that you have to get straightened out before you go. And you can't be understood, your situation can't be appreciated, until your family and friends, staring at you with embarrassed love, know—with an intimate, absolute knowledge—what your illness is like.[7]

A Short Bookshelf of Pathography

Andrews, Tom. *Cocaine Diary: True Confessions of a Reckless Hemophiliac.* New York: Harcourt Brace, 1998.

Brabner, Joyce, and Harvey Pekar. *Our Cancer Year.* New York: Four Walls Eight Windows, 1994.
Broyard, Anatole. *Intoxicated by My Illness.* New York: Clarkson Potter, 1992.
Donne, John. *Devotions upon Emergent Occasions.* London: Oxford University Press, 1987.
Job, The book of
Lee, Robert Mason. "The Man Who Was Saved by a Mouse." *Saturday Night*, April 21, 2001.
Mann, Thomas. *The Magic Mountain.* Translated by John E. Woods. New York: Vantage, 1995.
Rogers, Shelagh. "Speaking of Dying," in *Dropped Threads* 2. Edited by Carol Shields, Marjorie Anderson. Toronto: Vintage Canada, 2003.
Sacks, Oliver. *A Leg To Stand On.* New York: Simon and Shuster, 1984.
Updike, John. "At War with My Skin," *Self-Consciousness.* New York: Knopf, 1989.

A Very Useful Resource

The Literature, Arts, and Medicine Database, http://mchip00.med.nyu.edu/lit-med/lit-med-db

Notes

1. Brant Frayne, "My First Death," *Toronto Life*, September 2003, 66.
2. Robert Mayson Lee, "The Man Who Was Saved by a Mouse," *Saturday Night*, April 21, 2001.
3. Anatole Broyard, *Intoxicated by My Illness* (New York: Clarkson Potter, 1992), 38.
4. Sylvia Plath, "Tulips," *Collected Poems* (London: Faber and Faber, 1981), 160.
5. Tom Andrews, *Codeine Diary: True Confessions of a Reckless Hemophiliac* (New York: Harcourt Brace, 1998), 152.
6. Lee.
7. Broyard, 67.

Robert Maunder is a psychiatrist at Mount Sinai Hospital. His clinical practice and research focuses on problems of living with serious physical illness.

Elysium

Pamela Stewart

"My brain is for pleasure now," Peter says. He is pinned between the two women. They hold him in a sitting position on the bed. His wife, Rose, encircles his upper arm with one hand and supports his back with the other. Yvonne mirrors her actions. She is paid for her intimacy. His two daughters lean forward to hear. His voice has become as shrivelled as his body.

"That's good, Dad, only think about nice things," the oldest daughter, Susan, says.

"It's the body I don't trust," he says. "The body cheats you. It turns you into a jealous lover, always looking for signs of betrayal. The rest of the time it lulls you into a false sense of security. And when you're not looking, wham! You're the last to know. My body is divorcing me. Except for my teeth," he says, smiling at his reflection in the dresser mirror opposite the bed. "My teeth make me proud, and I'm taking them with me."

"Maybe it's the drugs making him like this," Rita, his other daughter, whispers to Susan. "Or maybe it's something no one knows about. Maybe the cancer has spread to his brain. Whatever it is, it's helping him. I mean, he seems almost happy."

"He can't be. He can't be happy to be dying," Susan says, "unless he's in denial. None of this would be happening now if he had quit smoking."

"He doesn't have lung cancer, Susan."

"Well this wouldn't be happening if he had eaten more fibre. Or something."

"You know it hasn't affected my hearing. I can hear you girls just fine," Peter says.

Rose gently pushes the two women toward the door. "Stop blaming your father for a disease. Everyone dies of cancer now. It doesn't matter what you eat or if you smoke. It's in the air, the water, the food. Stop lecturing. We all know smoking is bad, OK? Daddy doesn't deserve this. Now leave us so we can get him cleaned up."

"Sorry Dad, I didn't mean to imply . . ."

"It's OK, honey, I ask the same questions myself."

Yvonne helps her remove his damp pyjamas. They wash him gently.

He has a colostomy bag, and Yvonne takes care of it. The doctors had to remove a large section of the cancerous colon, followed by radiation and chemotherapy, but it was still too late. The cancer had spread to his liver.

"I don't want you looking at me, Rose. I've become so ugly. Let Yvonne do it. She's used to seeing people in this state. Sorry, Yvonne."

"Don't apologize. It's my job, and I like taking care of people."

Rose tells him he still looks like the man she married. She loves his damaged body.

"Call it like it is," he's says. "I'm rotting. You romanticize everything."

The women rub lotion into his skin. They turn him. Rose's hands echo the care she gave her three babies.

After they dress him, they help him into the chair next to the bed and cover him with a blanket.

"It's supposed to be the other way around. I should be carrying you."

"You did, remember? Over the threshold. In sickness and in health."

Peter always loved to lift Rose off her feet and carry her around. She was so tiny and light. He looks at the black-and-white photograph on the bedroom wall. They were still dating then. He is giving her a piggyback ride in the snow. They are smiling, and snowflakes cover their wool coats. He remembers shortly after his brother took the photograph, they fell backward into the snow, laughing and kissing each other, her rosy cheeks, plump with youth and cool against his face.

Rose opens the bedroom door and calls the others back.

Susan carries in clean sheets and lets her sister strip the bed of dirty sheets.

"I've brought these from outside where they've gathered the smells of the garden," she says.

She places a fresh sprig of lavender from the herb garden in the pillowcase.

When she leaves, Peter will throw it in the garbage.

Susan lives in a Martha Stewart world and sees everything, even illness, as a challenge to be overcome through home decor.

Earlier, she had brought in flowers and arranged them in containers, not noticing that he doesn't notice.

They fold him into a cloud. All white, feather bed, pillows, and duvet.

A ladybug crawls out of the pillowcase. They sit quietly and watch the drop of red until it flies away.

When they hear him snoring, they tiptoe out of the room.

"Every time he goes to sleep I'm afraid he won't wake up again," Rose says.

"I know. Like when you have a new baby and you watch it sleep so silently, you end up waking the baby to make sure it's still alive," Susan says.

The women sit around the kitchen table drinking tea and coffee and talking about babies. Rita's daughter is almost nine months pregnant with a son and lives in Montreal. Rita was supposed to be with her now. A part of her does not want her father to linger so she can be there for the birth of her grandchild.

"They are going to name the baby Pierre Michel, after Dad and Michael," she says.

Peter is alone in the bedroom dreaming about his son. Michael is driving a car and Peter is a passenger.

Michael says, "When you are driving, you are always heading into the future."

Peter watches the speedometer climb.

"Let's get there faster," Michael says.

He wakes confused. At first he thinks it is the day they told him his son was dead. Brain dead. They want to keep his body alive and remove the organs for donation. Rose, too distraught to make decisions, is sedated. He says yes. Michael had a donor card but they cannot find it. His body is sent to the funeral home after everything is removed. He wonders how he will get through it, picking out a casket, cremation or burial. That was ten years ago. He has thought of that day for over 3600 days now. He feels that the pain crept into his bones, slid into his bowels and remained there, causing the cancer that was now killing him. There would be no organ donation from him.

Colon cancer. Stage 4, also known as Dukes D. He asked his oncologist if it was named after John Wayne.

His doctor said, "Before you ask, it's a fallacy that John Wayne had forty pounds of impacted fecal matter in his bowels. No one can live like that. They never did an autopsy on him so no one knows how this rumour got started. People who do colonics, no doubt."

Rita comes into the room with a bowl of soup.

"Please, no more soup. I want something solid. Some meat."

"Daddy, you know your system can't handle real food anymore. Meat is what caused this."

Peter was allowed to eat whatever he felt he could tolerate, and it was too late to worry about such things now, but he went along for the most part with his family's care. She pushes the spoon toward his mouth and he bites her on the hand, not hard, but enough to indent marks on the skin.

"I have teeth," he says, "for masticating food."

Peter's smile was the best thing about him and he used it. His teeth were always perfect, white, and straight. He smiled naturally, and he found it opened people toward him. He smiles and falls back asleep.

Rita sits and eats the soup, then sneaks out of the room.

Peter wakes to see his dead son's daughter, Gina, sitting at the end of the bed. She fades into the darkness of the room dressed in her usual black. Her hair is dyed blue black and her eyes are rimmed in black liner.

"Look on the bright side: you won't have to get anything new for the funeral," he says to her.

"I'm going to wear red, because I know you like it. I've brought you a treat." She opens the foil wrapper of a burger with onions, tomato, relish, and mustard. She pulls a bottle of beer from her backpack and opens it and takes a sip then hands it to him. He doesn't question her, even though she is only sixteen years old.

"Don't tell," she says.

"It'll be our secret."

Other than Rose, Peter feels more comfortable with Gina than anyone. She knows something about death. She was six when her father died. She took it to heart when her mother told her that her father was still alive but in a different way, and that death is just another form of life. Her mother told her that one day she would be with her father when she gets to the other side, and she shouldn't be afraid, but it would be a long time and she should gather as many experiences as she can, so that when she gets there she will have lots of interesting stories to tell her dad.

Now Gina knows her grandfather will be seeing her father soon, and she has given him a book of poems she wrote for her father. They will put it in the casket and it will be burnt in the crematorium, and the spirit of that book will rise up as smoke in the air, mingling with the spirit of her grandfather.

In grade eight, Gina did a school project on Dia de los Muertos and practised her presentation on her grandfather, before they both knew he was sick. The people of Mexico were not afraid of death. They believed that during the Day of the Dead the departed family members will come to visit. Gina has a collection of Day of the Dead figurines, Calaveras. Little clay-and-wire skeleton people dressed in colourful clothes going about their lives. She has placed a Calaveras of a nurse on the bedside table to look after her grandfather.

They had decided they would travel together to Oaxaca next October for Day of the Dead, and there they would make an altar for Michael like the Mexicans do. They would decorate it with marigolds and chrysanthemums and have his favourite food and music and celebrate his life. They would eat candy skulls and sing and wait for his spirit to come.

Soon she would have one more reason to go. Peter provided the money for Gina and her mother, in his will, to take the trip together.

Gina made him feel free and alive. What others saw as morbid he found refreshing. She loved him intensely. He knew that and there was nothing frivolous in her behaviour.

"It's not my life flashing before my eyes at all," he says. "It's more like watching TV. Or a movie on the VCR. Stop, start, rewind."

"Skip the commercials," she says. "I hate it when you fall asleep watching TV. And the commercials sneak into your dreams. I think they're designed that way. They want it to become part of you."

"Yes."

Gina tells him that some other family members are here.

He says he wants to see them too, but he is tired and wants to sleep first.

The door in cracked open and two boys peek into the room.

"He's not in a coma is he?" one of them asks the other.

"He doesn't even seem that sick," another child says.

"Well he is. Mom said the doctors said he could die at home like he wants and that they couldn't do anything else for him except give him morphine and stuff."

"He did seem kind of out of it."

The sound of their voices overrides the fracas his cells are causing inside his body, and he is half awake.

He wafts in and out until Rose says, "I know you are in there."

"Jesus Christ has skin like porcelain and the blood looks so red dripping from the wounds. But he looks so clean and unblemished. His hair isn't greasy or tangled. Everything is like falling asleep in front of the TV," he says.

The doctor comes. Everyone leaves the room and he can't tell how much time has passed, but it doesn't seem to matter anymore. The doctor leaves.

It is night because it is dark and Rose is in the bed. She wanted to sleep on the cot next to the bed but he wants her there even if it causes pain.

"Let me rest my head on you." he says, "Oh, that's your breastless side."

"Breathless?" She feigns. "Yes. You still leave me breathless."

"No. I mean . . ."

"I know. It was supposed to be the other way around," she says. "I was supposed to go first."

He touches his hand to the scar and around her remaining breast. "Thank God it wasn't."

"I am space and time encased in skin. I am. Don't tell me I'm not," he says, when he wakes up in the middle of the night.

"I know you are."

"Take off our clothes."

She fumbles under the covers. It takes a long time.

Everything falls away. The one night stand he had when he was forty-five with a younger woman. He was out of town at a conference. Rose had not been feeling sexual for awhile. Drinks, a stranger, a hotel room, and he slipped. One time. He felt as if he had lost a part of himself with that woman and could never get it back. A strange strangling dark thing held him for days, but he did not tell Rose. He did not come home with flowers. He was cold to her for awhile as if he blamed her, and then one night she fell asleep in front of the television and he woke up alone in bed and realized how much he loved her. He went out to the living room and sat on the floor and looked at her face illuminated by the glow of a television preacher and then lifted her and carried her into bed.

The policeman at the door telling them their son had been killed in a car accident. The decision to divide his body as gifts to others who were dying.

The time he lost his job and didn't tell her for two weeks. Dressing for work every day and spending the day looking for a job, then sitting at the library.

The month after their youngest daughter left home, Rose checked into a motel because she didn't know how to be anything except a mother, and he was neglecting her as a wife. A cheap motel, because she didn't want to spend the money. She left him a note and told him she was OK so he wouldn't think something bad had happened to her.

He still believes she had an affair but chose to forgive her. She was alone for three days, and in that time watched television, knit him a sweater, and filled two notebooks with her fears about growing old and not knowing what to do with her life. When she came home, he took her to the Royal York. They had room service and champagne, though they couldn't really afford it.

She holds him and listens to his breathing.

Then he falls away from her. His father and mother lie naked on the bed. He sits between them, eight months old.

The boy reaches for his father's penis with his tiny hand. They laugh and his father picks the boy up and puts him in his crib. He watches them make love. He is inside his mother's womb and his father holds her tight.

He is in God's eye.

God looks down and he drops out like a tear. The tear lands on Rose's face as she

Kisses him goodbye.

Pamela Stewart's work has been published in literary magazines, most recently in Descant.

First Day on the Wards

Eileen Valinoti

I hugged my blue nurse's cape around me against the biting cold. On this frigid January morning, I was to begin my clinical nursing work in the hospital. It was still dark as I walked with three of my classmates the two blocks from the nurses' residence to St. Mary's Hospital, a decaying hulk of a building surrounded by tenements and factories. Gusts of wind blew through the streets scattering dried leaves and scraps of old newspapers into the freezing air.

In the deserted lobby of the hospital, we got on to a large ancient elevator that swayed and creaked its way slowly up to the female surgical unit where we had been assigned. On the walk to the hospital we had chattered like schoolchildren, delighting in the rustling sound of our starched blue-and-white uniforms, the silken feel of our nylon stockings against our legs, the swirl and drape of our heavy woolen capes with their red satiny linings and their high military style collars, emblazoned with our school's insignia. People on their way to the subway had looked dull and drab in their workaday clothes, the women in knotted kerchiefs, the men in dark caps, with flaps covering their ears. But now, as the elevator made its tortured ascent, everyone stared silently ahead. My stomach began to feel queasy from the rocking; in my excitement I had skipped breakfast. At last the elevator reached the fifth floor, shaking as it came to a sudden shrieking stop.

We stood in a circle at the nurses' station that adjoined a large open ward, waiting for our instructor, Sister Julianne, to give us our patient assignments. Some of us giggled nervously. A priest, his purple stole draped over his black cassock, rushed by.

"He's come to give the last rites," someone said in a frightened tone. A hush fell over our little group.

From the nurses' station, I could see clearly into the ward. The patients' beds were lined up against the wall, each one separated by flimsy green curtains. Some of the curtains were closed tightly, others wide open. The priest had disappeared into one of the shuttered cubicles, and I could hear him saying the droning prayers for the dying. The air was heavy with the odour of disinfectant.

"Ugh," a classmate whispered into my ear, "I can't stand that awful smell."

A woman whose face and head and arms were swathed in bandages walked unsteadily down the middle of the ward, leaning against a nurse. She must have been burned, I thought with horror. An agitated old lady in the first bed was banging a basin against the side rails. Her long white hair hung in disorder around her gaunt face, and her eyes seemed about to burst from their sockets with the force of her rage. What if Sister told me to take care of her? I fought back the impulse to run.

But instead I was assigned to a Mrs. Murphy, who had had her gallbladder removed a week before. She should have a complete bed bath, I was told. If time permitted, I was to take her for a short walk. All of us were to be finished and ready to meet Sister at the nurses' station at nine o'clock sharp.

"You have one hour," Sister said, peering at us intently over her glasses, "that's plenty of time."

Mrs. Murphy was an obese woman in her mid-fifties. Her grey hair was tangled and matted, and the strings of her short white hospital gown were undone. Rivulets of perspiration had pooled in the folds of her neck. She looked weary, but she smiled at me when I introduced myself, giving me some courage. She promptly forgot my name, deciding to call me "dearie."

I took the basin from her bedside table and went into the utility room at the end of the ward to fill it. A long line of student and graduate nurses had already formed. When my turn came, I worried over the temperature of the water, adjusting and readjusting the faucets from hot to cold and cold to hot and back again. In our nursing class, we had used a bath thermometer, but here in the real world, none was in sight. Behind me a senior student tapped her foot.

"Use your wrist," she said in an irritated voice.

Mrs. Murphy's bedside table was cluttered with get well cards, family photos, used cups and spoons. Her dentures rested in a cup of water. On the overbed table sat her empty breakfast tray. I had to deposit my basin next to it and clear everything away before I could even begin. Then I saw I had forgotten the bath blanket. Back again I went, past the long rows of beds to the linen closet. From behind the closed curtains of the dying patient, I could hear the prayers of the priest,

"Lord have mercy on her,

Christ have mercy on her."

In the next bed, a patient was retching and vomiting into a basin held by Sister Julianne. A wave of nausea came over me; I swallowed hard, averting my eyes. I looked at my watch; fifteen minutes had passed and I hadn't even started the bed bath. I felt myself in a race against the clock.

In the ward, people were perpetually coming and going: nurses were scurrying about taking temperatures and changing beds, doctors were making their rounds, aides were collecting breakfast trays and bedpans, patients were pushing themselves in wheelchairs or walking carefully, protective hands over their incisions, cleaning women were mopping the floors and dusting beds and shelves. A handyman stood on a ladder fixing a stuck window. The noise was constant. Radios blared traffic and weather reports, food and medication carts rumbled, trays banged, radiators hissed and gurgled, the heavy elevator door clanged as it opened and closed. Patients coughed, expectorated, groaned, called for the nurse, and sometimes shrieked. Their conversations were clearly audible as they cheered each other on: "You're doing good, Mary," a patient said to her neighbour, who was struggling to swallow a cup of thick, chalk-like liquid, following each gulp with a hand desperately clamped over her mouth.

Out of this chaos, an order began to emerge. I saw that the outraged white-haired lady had stopped banging her basin. She was sitting now in a chair, her hands folded in her lap over the wool blanket that covered her knees. Behind her, a nurse with a large powdered face and a no-nonsense look was braiding her hair. Other nurses were stripping beds of sodden sheets and covering them with crisp white ones, fragrant from the laundry. An air of efficient industry emanated from the nurses; I could sense the pleasure they took in their own brisk movements as they tucked in sheets and pulled them taut, plumped up pillows, and smoothed blankets and bedspreads. Breakfast trays were stacked and carted away, dirty linen vanished into a large hamper, the broken window was fixed and opened to breaths of fresh air. In my own small way, I felt part of this grand communal mission to set everything to rights, as I walked purposefully back to Mrs. Murphy, hugging the bath blanket, still warm and soft from the hospital dryer. She had dozed off, but she woke with a start when I approached.

There were many steps to follow when you gave a proper bed bath. First you covered the patient with the bath blanket, underneath which she could remove her gown. Next you fan-folded the top sheet and blankets to the bottom of the bed. You held the washcloth in your hand draped over your fingers like a mitt, so that the edges were folded down, not to irritate the patient's skin. Each body part was to be washed separately to avoid exposing more anatomy than necessary, preserving the patient's modesty.

We had practised all this with ease on our mannequin in the nursing arts classroom, but as I proceeded I soon saw that bathing a live human being was a different matter altogether. Mrs. Murphy moved restlessly about and often pushed aside the bath blanket. What if Sister made one of her impromptu inspections and saw a flagrantly exposed leg or arm, or worse? I could hardly confide in my patient, but she saw my look of alarm.

"It's so hot in here, dearie," she said apologetically.

We were taught that patients who were able should wash their own "private parts." But how did one express this and to a perfect stranger in the bargain? Sister said we should hand a clean washcloth to the patient and say, "You can finish the bath now."

But I was too embarrassed even to manage that, wordlessly handing the washcloth to Mrs. Murphy. She understood at once and began to scrub herself vigorously, not even waiting for me to hurry outside the curtains.

Down the ward I went again to the utility room for clean water. As I walked past the row of beds, I saw that the priest was gone, the curtains pulled tightly around the dying patient's bed. Underneath the curtains, I could see the bottom of Sister Julianne's white skirt. The nun seemed to be everywhere at once. From inside the cubicle, someone was sobbing. I felt a shiver of dread and quickened my steps.

It was time to wash Mrs. Murphy's back. But as she turned on her side, I saw a narrow rubber tube protruding from beneath her dressing. I heard myself gasp in shock. The tube was draining dark green bile into a large glass bottle on the floor. It was a miracle I hadn't knocked it over with my many nervous steps around the bed. And I had been so intent on covering up my patient, I had hidden the drain as well. Beads of sweat broke out on my brow.

"Never let a patient think you're nervous," we were told. I kept my smile intact as I wondered how I would get Mrs. Murphy out of bed tethered to her equipment. I poked my head outside the curtains to look for Sister Julianne. She was nowhere in sight. I thought with despair that now I would never finish on time if I finished at all.

A harassed nurse was pushing a medication cart down the centre of the ward. When she moved closer, I shut the curtains and stepped outside. "Can you help me?" I asked her timidly. Freshmen students were universally regarded as a nuisance.

"I'm very busy," she said frowning, but she left her cart and walked over to where I stood. I whispered my dilemma. Behind us, Mrs. Murphy waited trustingly.

"You just disconnect the tubing, clamp the drain and then tape it to her dressing." She fixed me with a look that said any fool knows that, and turned away to walk back to her cart.

I stood paralyzed with fright. I had no faith in my ability to deal with Mrs. Murphy's drain. What if when I handled it, it accidentally fell out? Or slipped in further? Which would be worse? I didn't know.

I prayed silently, "Holy Mother Mary, let her do it for me." Tears stood in my eyes.

The nurse looked anxiously at her watch.

"Oh, for God's sake," she said, sighing with exasperation and pulling a small metal clamp out of her pocket. She went into the cubicle, smiled at Mrs. Murphy, and in what seemed like one lightning movement, disconnected the tubing, clamped the drain, and taped it to the dressing, freeing Mrs. Murphy from her bottle of bile.

My knees went weak with relief. I finished washing Mrs. Murphy's back, rubbed it with alcohol, finishing off the job in a great cloud of Cashmere Bouquet Talcum Powder, and took her bathrobe from the hanger. She reached over to the bedside table for her dentures and put them in her mouth with a happy sigh. I asked her to hold onto me while I helped her into a chair, but she shook her head. "You're such a skinny little thing, dearie."

With great shuddering grunts and groans, she inched her way slowly to the edge of the bed, one hand behind her and the other holding her abdomen, bracing herself cautiously for the final descent—from the bed to the footstool to the floor, and at last, out of breath but victorious, to her seat in the hard straight-backed chair. When she was settled, I brushed her hair, glad to be doing something that had no procedure attached to it. I brushed and brushed, then Mrs. Murphy pinned it back from her face and into a tidy bun.

Now, her dignity restored and in her pretty blue robe, she no longer resembled a patient at all. She seemed brighter, more alert, even cheerful as she looked around at her surroundings, such as they were. For the first time I saw who she was—a sweet middle-aged lady, down on her luck (she was, after all, in that dreary open ward) putting on a brave face and making the best of things, humbly submitting to a fearful young girl like me.

She let me take her arm, and I took her for a triumphant little stroll around the ward, basking in Sister Julianne's approving smile. I looked at the big clock on the wall—it was five minutes before nine.

Eileen Valinoti is a registered nurse whose essays have appeared in popular magazines and nursing journals. Her story "Night Duty" was published in 2007 in The Healing Muse. *She lives in New Jersey with her family.*

On Call

Paul Whang

It's Friday and unfortunately I'm on call. Over the next twenty-four hours, I'll be sleep deprived. Patients will be transferred from the Emergency Department to the Operating Room, where everything—from broken bones and infected gall bladders to ruptured aneurysms—will be mended, removed, or repaired. The Labour and Delivery floor will call me for possible Caesarean sections and epidurals. In fact, any place in the hospital, from the Emergency Room to the patient wards—can call on me during a cardiac arrest. Just thinking about all these medical emergencies makes me feel tired.

And even if I do have the opportunity to sleep, it's a restless, agitated sleep—expectantly waiting for my pager to ring. I don't know what they'll call me for or why they'll need me, but I have to be ready. The unexpectedness and randomness of the events adds to my stress. I'll wake up frequently, suspicious of a pager malfunction, a missed call, or that I'm sleeping *too* well. It's a sad state to be in. When it is quiet and peaceful, I'm distressed by the serenity and become on edge again.

In fact, the pager becomes an accursed thing—the messenger that badgers and startles when you don't want to be disturbed: sitting on the toilet, occupied with an important clinical task, or just as your head snuggles into the soft pillow in anticipation of some blissful shut-eye.

After the seventh page in twenty minutes, I curse the pager, as if it were a malicious living creature waiting to taunt me at every opportunity. I feel like smashing it against the wall. I know my Freudian subconscious is truly at work, given the number of times the pager has *fallen* into the toilet—believe me, it can't be entirely accidental. But here's the sad thing: after I've dried it off, the damn thing *still* works, and the evil creature lives on.

Some hospitals have replaced pagers with cellphones. Other than the fact that cellphones may cost more, or that dead zones occur where cellphones are unreachable, I've got to admit I prefer the pager. Once a pager has stopped ringing, I can look at the display and then decide whether I want to respond to it right away. A ringing cellphone insists that I answer it and connect with someone immediately. The pager offers me a choice to *not* be instantly connected to someone.

I confess that when my pager indicates calls are coming from certain non-critical wards, I'll wait to be paged a second time before responding, giving myself a little extra rest. After all, the wards *have* often confused me with Dr. Wang (family doctor) or Dr. Wong (obstetrician), or Dr. Leong (gastroenterologist) in the past. Don't we all look the same, and have similar names? At least, that's my excuse.

My response to the pages deteriorates as the day progresses. Fatigue and irritation take their toll.

In the morning, it's "Hello. How are you? What can I do for *you*?"

By afternoon, it's "Anaesthesia on call. What's the problem?"

By late evening, it's "Yeah? *What is it?*"

As I grow older, I prepare for being on call with increasing dread. I laugh at myself now, recalling that years ago, when I first started practice, "On Call" would excite me. There was opportunity to apply your skills and knowledge, crystallized through years of study, to treat patients and overcome the challenges. It was like an adventure. Unfortunately, most of that excitement has been worn away, replaced with the feelings of heavy responsibility and fatigue. Hopefully, I can always retain the sense that I am doing some good for others.

When I'm on call, especially late at night, I'm called to various patient wards in the hospital. Each has its own characteristic atmosphere and feel. When entering the softly illuminated patient wards at night, my footsteps echo down the corridors. Sometimes, it feels like entering the sanctuary of a monastery. It's a subdued atmosphere, where every effort is made to give peace and quiet to the patients—patients who have had to endure endless rounds of tests and procedures during the day and who are now seeking the solace and serenity of the night. When arriving at the nursing desk late at night, we try to preserve this peace and calm and speak in whispers.

In contrast, if you're called to the emergency room in a large urban hospital, it's truly like a television episode of ER—loud and chaotic, with paramedics constantly arriving with injured and sick patients. Seriously ill patients are hustled to resuscitation rooms. The less seriously ill are made to sit endlessly in the overcrowded waiting room, hoping to be next in line to see the Emergency Room doctor. The stress level on the nurses and doctors is very high. With some people, tension boils just below the surface.

At times like this, I often feel that I've entered an area of the hospital where the idea of camaraderie is thrown out the window. For example, I ask, "Could you tell me where the order forms are?" Response from the ER nurse, with glaring eyes, "Can't you see I'm busy?! *Get it yourself!*"

After 11 p.m., I think they become zombies. Sometimes they don't even acknowledge me or just give me a blank stare.

The Labour and Delivery Ward, or, as it is occasionally referred to, "The House of Scream," is another story. Upon entering, I'm usually greeted by the cries of women in the midst of painful labour. Of course, I don't mind inserting epidurals in mothers-to-be during the day. But what is occasionally bothersome occurs when the mother was asked if she wanted an epidural while the labour pains were mild and infrequent—yet she refused to even consider this midway through her labour. She wanted to proceed "naturally." Much later, I'm called back at the wretched hour of 3 a.m. The patient's cervix is well dilated, with severe contractions occurring every two minutes.

The challenge now is to try to insert a large, sharp, and potentially paralyzing epidural needle into the back of the labouring woman, centimetres from the spinal cord, in between the contractions and screams of pain—and to do so on a moving target. You can understand why I'm a little miffed with her earlier decision to wait.

It's highly stressful for the new dad-to-be. His face is usually filled with perspiration and panic as he sympathetically anticipates and experiences each contraction with his partner. Many times the poor man is the focus of all the rage, frustration, and pain that the woman experiences: "*You* did this to me . . . How can *you* understand what I'm going through!

. . . You'll *never* understand!" I've heard curses and abuses hurled at the poor guy—who wants only to "be there" and be supportive to his partner.

I've changed my routine of allowing the father to stay and hold the hand of his partner while I insert the epidural. In my mind's eye, I've too often seen his ashen face, his eyes rolling up. He moans that he doesn't feel too well, just before he faints with a dull thud beside the bed. The nurses and I have to try to catch him early, before he loses consciousness and becomes another casualty.

"Honey, Honey, are you OK?" the woman asks, trying to get a glimpse of her partner, as his head starts to sink towards the floor.

"He's going to be OK. Just needs a little fresh air," says the Labour Room nurse, as she helps the disorientated man to his feet.

"He's OK, isn't he?" she again asks.

"He'll be fine! I'm just going to help him out of the room. Now you just concentrate on being still with the doctor!" says the nurse, as she assists the man out of the room.

"Now just be still. Don't move! I'm about to put the needle in," I remind her, again for the fifth time.

"*Ow, ow*! I can feel another contraction coming! I *can't* be still!" She screams for the sixth time as she sways.

Sigh. Here we go again, I think to myself. And so it goes.

AFTER YEARS of "On Call," having met so many people who face sudden illness, it's easy to automatically classify them and believe I'm able to predict their behaviour. But "On Call" teaches you to abandon your biases and judge each person as an individual.

Mr. B. was one of these people. On this night, the surgeon called to say that an operation was needed to remove a bullet from his thigh—a drug deal gone bad. Mr. B. was stable and was being prepared for surgery.

"By the way, he's got no health insurance," the surgeon added, in a tired and frustrated tone, indicating that we would be providing charity medical service this late night. I would have go to Mr. B. directly for payment, if I ever hoped to be paid. More often than not, in a big city hospital, you resign yourself to the reality that even if you're fatigued, hungry, and it's late at night, you will not be paid for some of your services.

Each year, more and more people enter the city, working under the radar, seeking anonymity. For various reasons, they shun and reject the support systems offered—like health insurance.

If the person is destitute, or clearly just eking out a living, you just accept the realities of the situation and do your job. But, very occasionally, you sense that some may have the means to pay for health services, and so you inquire about compensation. What risk is there in asking?

With low expectations, I went down to the emergency room to visit Mr. B.

As I approached a room in the distant area of the Emergency Department, I was stopped at the doorway by two human towers dressed in black—one who resembled Andre the Giant and the other who looked like the brother of Shaq O'Neil. "What do you want?" one growled, glaring eyes threatening me.

"I'm looking for Mr. B.," I squeaked, regretting more and more my decision to come.

From within the room, a raspy voice called out, "Let him in."

As I entered, two very sleek, scantily dressed, and stunningly beautiful women sat cross-legged on either side of the bed—their miniskirts leading my eyes along silken thighs, towards the mesmerizing curves of their torsos. And sitting between them, with a large bandage wrapped around his right thigh, was a small man in dark glasses. Cascades of gold jewellery glistened around his neck and shining rings were on his fingers. I drew a large breath, gathered courage, and said, "Mr. B., I understand that you don't have any insurance, and I've just come here to tell you that there is a charge for anaesthetic services."

He regarded me silently for some time and then took his glasses off. His face was not at all what I expected. It revealed a thoughtful man, his quizzical eyebrows accenting brown eyes that expressed a quiet intelligence, his breathing slow and measured, lips pursed in thought as he studied me.

And he knew me. He understood my uneasiness, my attempt to obtain payment from a drug dealer who doesn't operate by the normal rules—a man who didn't have to pay, who could blow me off at any time, and, with a gesture, could have the giants eject me from his room.

He suddenly straightened up, sat erect, and decreed, "Don't worry. Mr. B. is good for it. I'm a man of my word." And as he said this, his face was a mixture of defiance and honour, while a thumb in a clenched fist pointed at his chest.

I thanked him and, with much relief, rushed out of the room.

The surgery proceeded smoothly.

To be frank, I really didn't believe that Mr. B. would pay me. There are no practical options to seek compensation in these situations. Credit agencies have no sway. Letters from lawyers emphasizing the serious legal consequences that would follow non-payment are, of course, laughable.

However, the next day, I gathered my courage and decided to make my way to Mr. B's room after surgery. Again standing on either side of the entrance were the large bodyguards. I asked for admission, and his voice ushered me in. The two beautiful women were nestled beside him as he recovered in bed—still breathtakingly exotic and beautiful. I asked him how he felt. Everything was fine, and, according to him, I had done a good job.

There was silence. He then looked me straight in the eyes, and asked, "How much?"

I quoted him the fee. He slowly reached into the pocket of his embroidered robe and pulled out a very large roll of $100 bills. He slowly counted, then handed me the money.

I thanked him again, and as I started to leave, he spoke, his voice full of dignity and pride, "I told you not to worry, Mr. B. is a man of his word."

I HAVE TO ADMIT, I sometimes become jaded by illness and even death. This is not a response uncommon among people who are involved in high-stress, life-and-death situations. It's a defence mechanism that allows you to distance yourself from the sadness. Getting personally involved with every patient is exhausting. Like firemen, policemen, and other health-care workers, we depersonalize the situation. Conversations are filled with grim humour. The whole situation becomes coldly clinical.

However, events occur sometimes that re-humanize us, creating a strong connection to certain patients. These episodes happen, seldom during the operation itself, but just before and after.

4 p.m. The orthopaedic surgeon has been asked to fix the broken hip of Mrs. Krakow. He tells me that even though she's only fifty years old, she has breast cancer that has spread throughout her body. The cancer

has invaded her liver, causing metabolic poisons and bile to accumulate in her blood, so that her skin and even the whites of her eyes are stained yellow. The metabolic toxins make her confused. Cancer has spread to her bones, making them so brittle that a simple fall can cause her hip to break like a toothpick.

He tells me this to reassure me that Mrs. Krakow's hip will not be fixed tonight, or *any* night in the future. He considers her too high a risk for surgery: her body cannot metabolize drugs; her risk of significant blood loss during surgery is great; and she is confused. Finally, the fact is that she will die soon.

As he walks away, my pager rings. It's Mrs. Krakow's family doctor. He apologizes for paging me but explains that, despite her condition, he still would like me to see her and assess if there is even a small possibility that her hip can be repaired. I reluctantly agree to see her, though I am secretly in agreement with the assessment of the surgeon.

On the ward, a review of Mrs. Krakow's medical records verifies the bleak picture. Her room is at the end of the old section of the hospital. As I trudge down the corridor to her room, I hear my steps resonate off its bleached walls.

Her room is dark, small, and stuffy. A very small window faces the brick wall of the adjacent building. I'm surprised she is not lying in bed, but instead is sitting up, despite what must be terrible pain in her broken hip. She is struggling to gaze out the window from her bed. As she turns her head, I see that her face is large and puffy, the result of steroids used to slow the cancer. The hair on her scalp is thin and wispy, and there are bald areas scattered throughout her scalp—the signs of futile chemotherapy regimes. She has large, yellow-stained eyes that almost bulge out of her face. In the corners of her eyes I can see the reflection of the overhead lights. I realize her eyes are filled with tears.

I explain to her that I've come to assess her candidacy for surgery. As the tears glisten, she interrupts me and speaks forcefully, her voice a mix of determination and urgency. I quickly realize that she is not confused at all. She is fully aware of her situation.

I'm caught off guard as she pleads to have the surgery. She knows that she has terminal cancer, that the cancer has spread throughout her body, and that she only has a short time to live. She has no immediate family. She has vowed to get out of the hospital and be as independent as she possibly can be.

Before her accident, she was outside every day, despite her weakness and fatigue. She would go shopping every day. It was during one of these outings to the supermarket that she fell and broke her hip. Now, she is a prisoner in this room. Her only view of the outside world has been the bricks of the adjacent building from the small window in her room.

For the last two days, she had been evaluated by specialists and she realizes that she had only a small chance to have surgery. I can see the desperation in her eyes as she pleads with me for the surgery, despite the high risks. She tells me she does not want to die in this bed. She wants to be able to walk outside again and feel the sun.

I try to reassure her that I will attempt to convince the surgeon to perform the operation. I am aware that she is a high-risk patient and that she may not survive the surgery or the recovery period.

As I make my way from the ward, I feel so ashamed. I had come to assess Mrs. Krakow, like a medical bureaucrat, to certify the hopelessness of her situation and deny surgery— in effect, to sign her death certificate. She had ripped the cold clinical mask from my face. She had nothing to hide—no hidden agendas, no deception, just the stark reality of her dilemma—a person requesting one last chance for happiness before death.

But the images of this poor lady, facing death and trapped in a miserable room, desperate to get out—her face and eyes, her thoughts and voice echoing in my head— has affected me deeply. She has to be helped.

1:00 a.m. Dr. Bose is calling me. He is a burly man in his early sixties. His face has begun to show the effects of long surgical career—furrowed eyebrows and permanent creases between his eyes, a reflection of his cynicism after years of practice. He is a stubborn man. He would definitely go left if you were to say, "Go right." His gruff demeanour is in no way a reflection of his surgical skill—his large hands move with the delicacy and grace of a skilled painter, every movement a marvel of precision and purpose. He's had years of experience as a surgeon and probably has seen every operative scenario imaginable.

Everyone knows that Dr. Bose will be retiring soon. His practice is slowly winding down and he is counting the days of "On Call" left to do, like a prisoner counting the remaining days of incarceration. His operating philosophy is simple: avoid surgery if at all possible, if it has the potential to get you into trouble.

"Hi Paul. I just want to get your opinion about this guy that the intensive care doc is trying to get me to operate on ... and I don't want to operate on him! The patient's name is Fallis, and he was operated on two weeks ago for a perforated intestine (literally, a hole in the gut). He's got a terrible history—diabetes, drug addiction, heavy smoker with lung disease, recurrent pancreatitis. He was doing fine and was let out on a day pass today, and now he's suddenly had to come back in the hospital. He's in Intensive Care being ventilated and they're having trouble keeping his oxygen levels up and his blood pressure —it's only about seventy and he's on big-time drugs just to keep it there. His blood sugars are way out of whack, and his kidneys aren't working. He's a very high risk for surgery, don't you think?"

I tried to focus and shake the fatigue out of my eyes. It had already been a very long day of call, with numerous cases that seemed to go nonstop throughout the night.

"Yeah, I think he'd definitely be a high-risk patient, with a risk of dying on the table!" I said.

"That's what I wanted to hear! OK, thanks. I'll tell the intensive care doc that there's no way I'm doing this case. Bye."

I sat down thinking. "Fallis, Fallis? I remember that name!" Suddenly it all came back to me. Two weeks ago I had worked with another surgeon who cut out the leaking hole in Mr. Fallis's intestine and reattached the cut ends together. I remembered how Mr. Fallis had entered the operating room that day. He was only forty-nine years old, and the corroding effects of years of drug abuse, poor nutrition, and life as a street person had taken its toll and punished his body. He was rail thin and had the look of a starving man twenty years older—hollowed cheeks, ghost-like complexion, and thinning white hair. The ribs on his chest resembled those of a cadaver, and heavy cigarette stains coloured the fingers of his right hand. I recalled the pain and fear in his eyes as we transferred him to the operating table. We tried to reassure him that everything would work out fine. The surgery proceeded uneventfully and it seemed to us that, with his gut fixed, he could perhaps eventually recover. But given his poor physical status, the recovery would be very long and difficult.

What I recall most was the notation on the computer as I reviewed his medical history prior to surgery: "Has a thirteen-year-old son."

It wasn't standard practice to list personal information like that (in a list of medical problems). But for some reason the person inputting this information decided to tell us about this man's son. It changed my viewpoint of Mr. Fallis—not just a lifelong drug abuser and street person, but in fact a man with a family. It also brought things into personal perspective—I have a thirteen-year-old son.

I wanted to know how he had become so quickly and critically ill again. And so I called the intensive care doctor working that night. I was reassured when I found that Dr. Fine was working that night. A compact figure with a reassuring, kind face, his understated and quiet manner veiled an imposing clinical acumen and wry sense of humour. There are good and bad doctors. David is definitely in the "good" camp, an excellent diagnostician and clinician. I knew that any patient would have the best possible care under Dr. Fine.

He is also a reasonable person. He knows when to treat patients with high-powered drugs and techniques to try to save them—or when to gently discuss with their relatives that they are too sick for heroic measures. He knows when it would be merciful to let someone go peacefully.

"David, what's going on with Mr. Fallis?" I asked.

"Well, he was out today for the first time since his initial operation. It's his wife's birthday. He was walking when he suddenly had abdominal pain and collapsed. He's got a thirteen-year-old son, you know."

"I know," I replied, reminded again of my own son. "I was involved with his initial surgery."

Dr. Fine paused. "I put a tube down his airway and have got him on the ventilator. I've got Levophed infusing into him to maintain his blood pressure. He's very sick but I've got him stabilized best as I can. I really think his anastomosis [the previous intestinal repair] has fallen apart."

If this was the case, it would mean that feces were now leaking directly into Mr. Fallis's abdomen and blood. The highly toxic bacteria from the bowel would create a septic infection in the bloodstream with toxins affecting all organs of the body. The lungs would fail to oxygenate the blood, the kidneys would start to shut down, and the heart would fail.

"If that's the case," I said, "then his only hope is to get that anastomosis fixed. Is that what you think David?"

"Yes," replied Dr. Fine. "Andy's refusing to operate, saying that Fallis is too sick to withstand the operation. Andy doesn't want to kill him in order to try and fix problems that I can't 100 per cent say is the cause. Andy says Fallis could be septic from another source, like pneumonia, and he could have recurrent pancreatitis as well."

I was immediately filled with guilt. Andy had called me earlier and gave me only the basic sketch of Mr. Fallis's grave condition, not mentioning the possible post-surgical breakdown of the anastomosis. I had agreed with him, that there was a high possibility of intra-operative death, given the clinical story he'd given me. But I felt I had been misled to concur with Andy's desire not to get involved.

On the other hand, I understand the enormous responsibility and pressure he must have felt as the surgeon on call. This decision was the ultimate life-or-death Catch-22. Should the surgeon operate in order to save a life, knowing that the stress of the operation may kill the patient? Or should the surgeon wait until the patient is "optimized" and stabilized, knowing that optimization may be insufficient or never occur? In this case, the patient may die before the operation.

"Should I call another surgeon to operate?" I could hear the hint of desperation and exasperation in his voice.

"No, you just can't do that, David. You *know* that Andy's on call and is the responsible physician. Anyway, the other surgeons would repeat what I just said and refuse to come in. And you know Andy—if you were to try to push him, he'd just dig in his heels and you would get nowhere!"

There was a long pause and then a sigh from Dr. Fine. "Well, I'll just have to stabilize him the best I can, and hope that he hangs on until the next surgeon begins his call. Thanks for calling, Paul."

I looked at my watch. It was 1:30 in the morning. The next surgeon would begin call at around seven, after receiving a report from Andy about patients seen during his shift.

At 7:15 I went to the cafeteria. I definitely needed a strong cup of coffee to stay awake. Throughout the early morning, the Labour and Delivery ward had kept me busy with requests for epidurals. Any thoughts of Mr. Fallis had long since been pushed back during the busy hours of the morning. But as I poured coffee, Dr. Fine walked in to the cafeteria. For a brief moment we glanced at each other and then looked away. Seeing Dr. Fine immediately reminded both of us about the frustration and helplessness of our earlier conversation. We then both walked towards the cashier with our coffees.

"How is Mr. Fallis doing?" I asked.

His weary face met mine. He hesitated, and then in a soft voice replied, "He died around 4:30 this morning."

"Oh," I replied, as faint hope left me—replaced with guilt-tinged anger and disappointment I could feel rising within me.

"Too bad he just couldn't hang on a bit longer. The operation might have saved him."

"Yes, it might have," I replied.

There was a pause, and then we parted. And all the while, as I trudged up the stairs to the locker room, wearily pulled off my OR greens, and even as I left the hospital, I could only think about Mr. Fallis and his thirteen-year-old son.

Paul Whang graduated from the McMaster Medical School anaesthesia program. This excerpt is from his book, Operating Room Confidential, *which was published in 2010 by ECW Press.*

Making Images

Arthur Robinson Williams

The body anchors the Self in the physical world. A locus of materiality, it is the body that places us before the eyes of others, both vulnerable and intimidating. Yet for all that the body reveals of the Self, much of how we exist in the world eludes our fleshed corporeality.

Trans individuals (by which I mean to refer to transgendered, transsexual, and gender-variant individuals) by virtue of their trans status are familiar with such a notion, that the body can represent but also sabotage—whether through brutal honesty or gross betrayal—the inner Self.

Photography adds additional layers to lived representation and the embodiment of the Self. Through the hands of another's lens, the body takes on additional burdens of meaning and the true inner Self is further obscured by creeping layers of film.

My work with transfolks is meant to explore this tension between body and Self. Similar to illness, one's trans status may realize a gulf between the Self one is able to be and the Self one yearns to know. How to represent such loss and desire in a photograph becomes a collaboration. Much like an ideal clinical encounter, the image constructed is a partnership between the actors involved.

Similar to my medical training, photography has affected my approach to patient care. Having spent eight years travelling across the country and around the world photographing marginalized communities, I have come to appreciate how the process of making images is itself tantamount to the final prints.

For the participants with whom I have worked, the act of making a

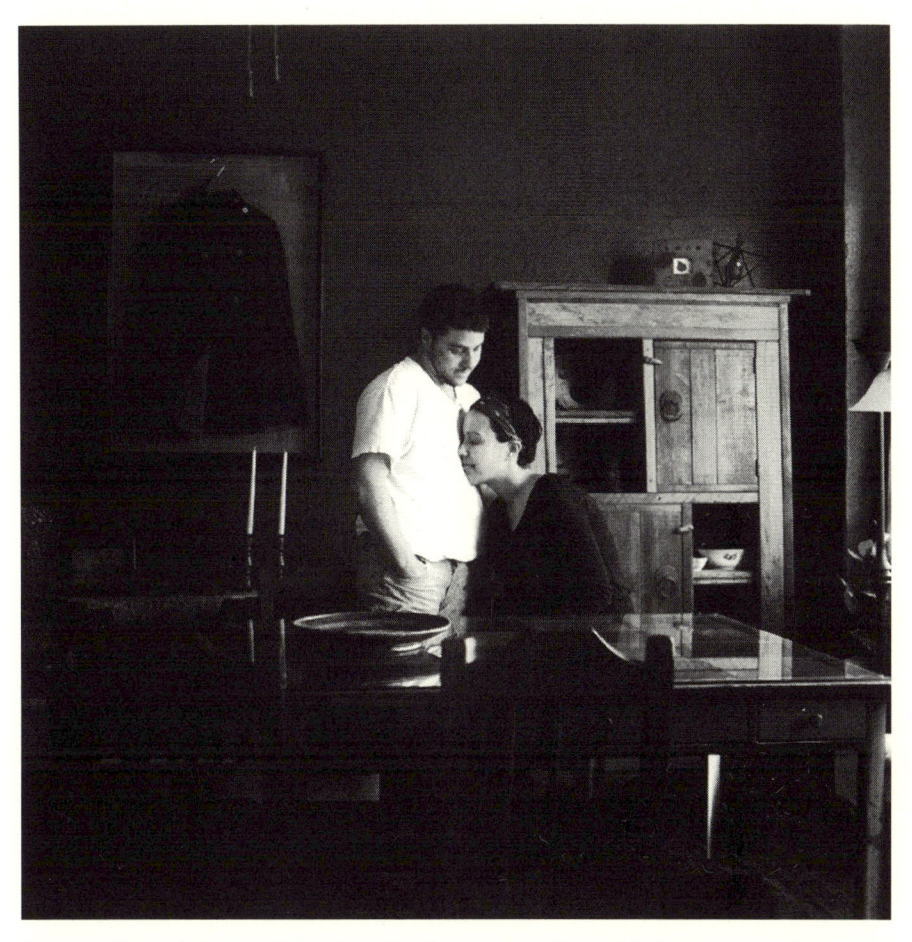

Dane and Erin. "There are always things I think people would change about their bodies. I know no man whose chest is big enough, hairline is stable enough, abs are eight-pack enough. I don't think I am above all these influences. I wish I were taller and I wish my chest were without scars. Although they are fading slowly, my scars are pretty prominent."

photograph has become—should be—as cathartic as the knowledge that the images will eventually reach a broader audience and as profound as the impact of the images upon viewers. For patients, likewise, the journey toward diagnosis and treatment may have as marked an impact on their latter years as their medical condition and/or disease state.

Ultimately the impact of images upon others is as much a reflection of the content of the photographs as it is revelatory of the viewer's own

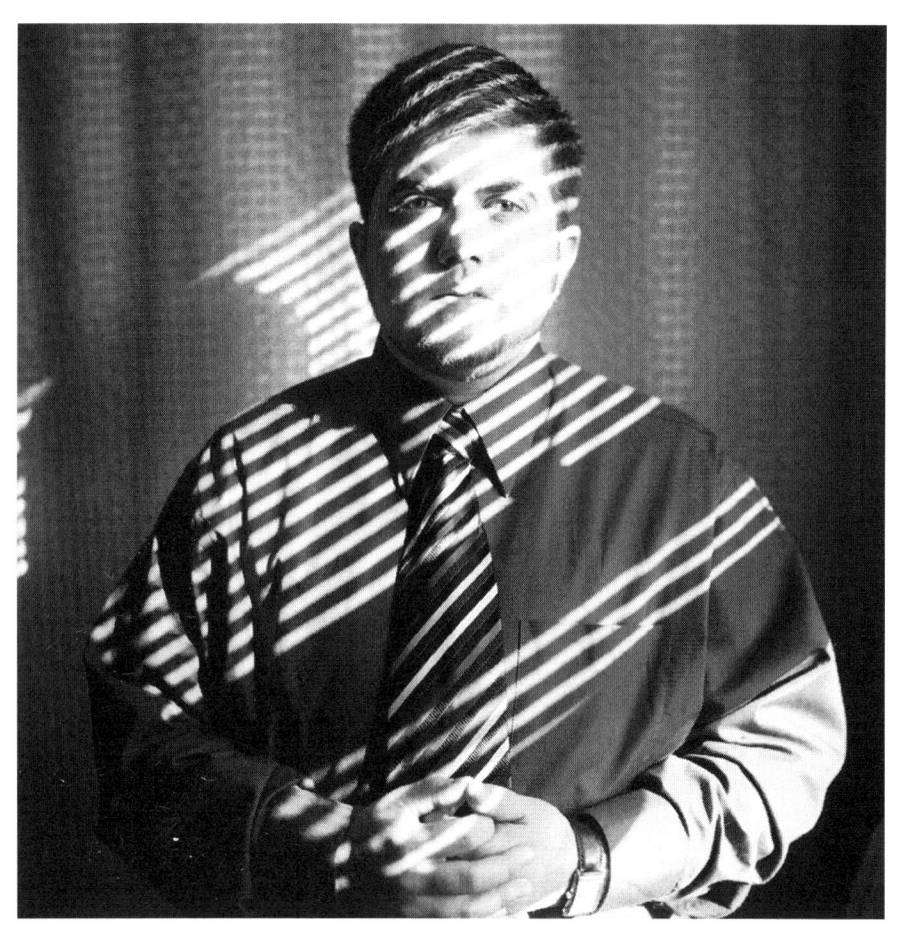

Jake. "I gained confidence in my ability to pass, not only physically but socially as well. From there I started going to gay bars—not to hook up, but just to be there, to be around gay men, again, to be in gay space that I felt safe navigating. I liked letting gay men flirt with me. It made me feel validated in my gender."

embodied Self. The viewer beholds the image, the viewer's corpus a conduit for the Self's accession of meaning-making. With regard to images of trans individuals, the viewer's own flesh is called into question. The empathic response to the loss and desire of another is itself the inward reflection upon who we are able to be and the Self we would one day like to know.

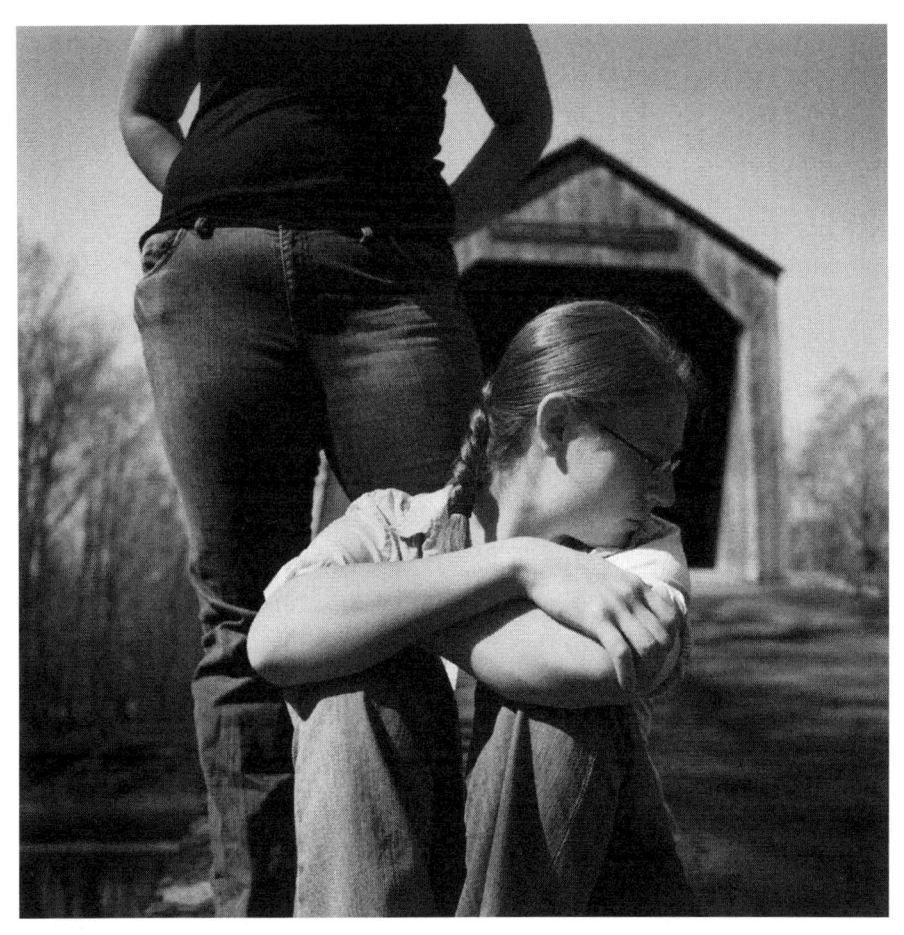

Allie and Mel. "The first major change came when I started on estrogen and anti-androgens. For the first time in my life, I felt right. I knew that soon the male body I possessed would be male only in certain ways."

Arthur Robinson Williams is a medical student at the University of Pennsylvania School of Medicine. Williams studied photography at Princeton with Emmet Gowin, Mary Berridge, and Lois Conner. His work can be found at www.MyRightSelf.org.

Ars Medica: A Journal of Medicine, the Arts and Humanities, is a biannual literary journal, started in 2004, that explores the interface between the arts and healing, and examines what makes medicine an art.

Founding Editors: Allison Crawford, Rex Kay, Allan Peterkin, Robin Roger, and Ronald Ruskin
Editor: Pier Bryden
Contributing Art Editor: Stephen Smart
Assistant Managing Editor: Terrence Sooley

Please visit the journal's website: http://ars-medica.ca/About.html

Ars Medica is published by University of Toronto Press. To subscribe, or to order single copies of the journal, visit the website of UTP Journals: http://www.utpjournals.com/